Injury Prevention and Rehabilitation in Sport

Ross Bennett

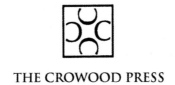

THE CROWOOD PRESS

First published in 2015 by
The Crowood Press Ltd
Ramsbury, Marlborough
Wiltshire SN8 2HR

www.crowood.com

British Library Cataloguing-in-Publication Data
A catalogue record for this book is available from the British Library.

ISBN 978 1 84797 957 5

Acknowledgements
I would like to say a huge thank-you to my wife Lucia and all my family for their continued support for my career so far. I would also like to acknowledge all lecturers and work colleagues who have contributed to my learning over the years, and have helped me mould a personal philosophy within strength and conditioning/sports science. I hope you all enjoy the book.

Disclaimer
The author and publishers of this book do not accept any responsibility whatsoever for any error or omission, nor any loss, injury, damage, adverse outcome or liability suffered as a result of the use of the information contained in this book, or reliance upon it. Since some of the training exercises can be dangerous and could involve physical activities that are too strenuous for some individuals to engage in safely, it is essential that a doctor be consulted before training is undertaken.

Typeset by Sharon Dainton Design
Printed and bound in India by Replika Press Pvt Ltd

CONTENTS

ABOUT THE AUTHOR

Ross Bennett was originally an aspiring football player registered with a number of Premier League football clubs as a youth team player but after injury and lack of progression he decided to enter the academic world. In 2008 he enrolled on the BSc Strength and Conditioning Sciences degree programme at St Mary's University, Twickenham. While in his second year Ross was offered a part-time internship at Chelsea FC Academy and was subsequently offered a part-time role at the club.

He spent four years at Chelsea, during which time he completed an MSc in Human Performance (Sports Science) at Brunel University. Both his dissertation research papers won best research poster at the annual UKSCA conference two years in a row (2011 and 2012).

Following a brief spell at the Aspire Centre in Qatar working with one of the national teams, he returned to the UK and currently heads the Strength and Conditioning team at Queens Park Rangers FC Academy.

INTRODUCTION

This current textbook outlines and discusses key areas that are essential for the reduction of injury when working with athletes on a daily basis or part time, depending on the level and age of the athlete. It will look at varying aspects and ideas in isolation to reduce injury rates, as well as providing ongoing personal philosophies of mine, which will run throughout the chapters. Although increasing performance isn't the priority of this current textbook, it will become apparent that the two often go hand in hand, with either a direct stimulus to both, or providing a stable base for performance enhancement, while having the underlying aim of reducing potential for injury.

The book's content combines scientific research findings, critical review of the current literature, and my personal experience working in the field of strength and conditioning at elite level. Some areas will have a greater focus on research; others that lack direct research will adopt an approach based on ideas that I have assimilated as a practising strength and conditioning coach. It must be noted, however, that although other concepts may be based on my current experience in the field, I do not claim to be the sole inventor of these techniques; instead my practice frequently involves generic modalities that have been implemented by many practitioners previously. The aim of this textbook is to provide a structure in which the reasons why these modalities should or should not be prescribed are discussed. Furthermore, to summarize and tie together all the injury prevention techniques, a diagrammatic structure is given at the end of Chapter 9 to link all the modalities together, highlighting their importance in injury prevention.

The rehabilitation section (Chapter 10) explores techniques available to the practitioner when an athlete is immobile and during recovery and rehab. It is not my intention to tread on the toes of the physiotherapists or sports therapists in clinical injury prevention: some interesting tips are given on how to assist the work of the therapist and possibly bridge the gap between rehab and fully functional sports training without restriction.

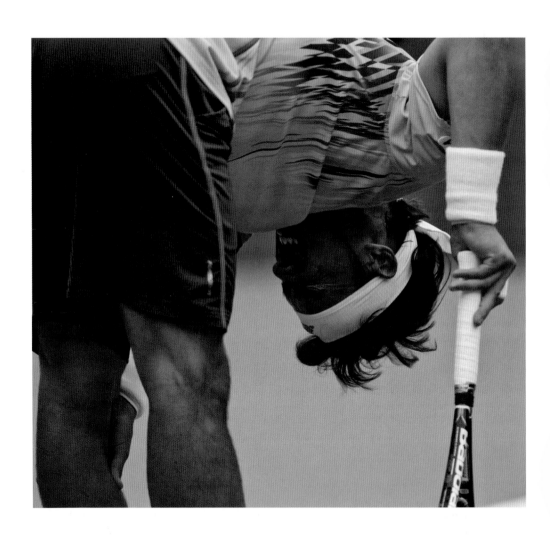

1 THE IMPORTANCE OF MAXIMAL STRENGTH

It is an often neglected consideration in strength and conditioning that a well-constructed strength programme can act as a key factor in injury prevention as well as a tool for performance enhancement. Increasing the strength of key musculature and connective structures causes an increase in their integrity and robustness. This in turn enables larger acute forces or greater volume and an increasing training stimulus to be applied without a potential breakdown. Furthermore, depending on the anatomical region of strength increase, this will elicit injury prevention benefits by increasing the stability of a joint. For example, strengthening the hamstrings will directly result in increased stability of the knee joint, thus illustrating the important role the hamstrings play in stabilizing the knee (Olsen *et al.*, 2005). Therefore, stronger hamstrings in particular will in turn reduce direct hamstring injuries such as tears, and consequently knee injuries, especially reducing injuries involved in rotation of the knee. (The importance of posterior chain strength and benefits will be explained in greater detail in a later section of this chapter.)

It may seem that this chapter is placed out of order in injury prevention programme design, as there are essential components of reducing injury that might be prescribed prior to strength training. For example, an athlete's ROM (range of movement) and stability around particular joints could be a focus prior to heavier strength training, and a later chapter within this book will specifically discuss the importance of corrective exercise to the athlete. However, this chapter was selected to appear first, as I believe (particularly in the sport in which I work – football) maximal strength is often neglected and misunderstood, including the benefits it can have in reducing injury rates.

Many practitioners within the field of strength and conditioning are over-cautious when applying strength training programmes to athletes, either because they are concerned for their safety, or they are worried that it might create a physiological adaptation of hypertrophy that is deemed detrimental to athletic performance. To combat this, a strength development programme is given in this chapter, which enables a modified long-term athletic development (LTAD) programme to ensure a safe and steady progression to increased strength. Guidelines are given in this chapter to create strength adaptation without necessarily causing an increase in any unwanted hypertrophy.

A progression/continuum for strength development is given below. Note that coaches and sports scientists will not always have access to athletes as young as nine, so the following steps can be applied and adapted to athletes at any age. LTAD is examined in much greater detail in Chapter 8 (Maturing and Youth Athletes).

STAGE 1 (AGE 9–12): INTRODUCTION TO FUNDAMENTAL MOVEMENT PATTERNS

Create mobility drills that will ensure an athlete is able to generate full ROM. Body weight exercises are essential; ensure that movement occurs with no dysfunction or compensation. If you have access to players at this age group, then this stage is essential and conforms to the high flexibility and ROM an athlete has at this age (this naturally decreases as chronological age increases). The aim is to provide a wide range of exercises, to broaden an athlete's skills set and to challenge them from a motor skill development point of view.

STAGE 2 (AGE 13–14): INCREASING MOTOR CONTROL

Still prescribing a combination of bodyweight and loaded exercises, exercise prescription should be restricted to those that will be more essential for functional strength development, although variation at times is essential for psychological/physiological benefit. A list of key exercises and the benefit of each one will also be included in this section. We can now start to increase the intensity and volume a bit

more, but ensure the movement is under good control. Take extra care when working with this age group: as they go through greatest peak height velocity phases (growth spurt) some athletes can experience movement issues or difficulties. This phase should also start to look at individuals who need specific ROM or stability work. Commonly, supplementary glute strength and ankle ROM training is required to enhance movement quality.

STAGE 3 (AGE 15–16): HIGH VOLUME LOAD TIME (WORK CAPACITY STRENGTH)

After previous technical phases and motor control work, it's time to increase the intensity in the gym. Based on previous experience, keeping volume relatively high post growth spurt and gradually increasing intensity seems to bridge the gap between motor control phases and general maximal strength work. Remember: if the load is higher than what the athlete is used to or has lifted before, an overload is created, which is essential for adaptation. If you are fortunate enough to be working with your athletes from a younger age, at this stage of their development there is often a natural increase in circulating hormones such as testosterone to assist further neurological gains and is thus an appropriate time to apply strength work. However, all athletes develop and mature at different times, and some may still have late growth issues as they go though PHV phases. Athletes go through their optimal strength/weight gaining phase approximately 18 months after PHV. It is therefore the responsibility of the coach and practitioner to assess the appropriate timing for the implementation of this phase.

Stage 4 (age 17+): TRADITIONAL MAXIMAL STRENGTH PHASE

After the three previous phases, your athlete should now be technically and physically competent, and can be prescribed a well-constructed traditional periodized strength programme to maximize their strength over a period of time. A guide to recommended repetitions is given; there will also be a section on periodization later in this textbook to demonstrate the importance of volume and intensity and how it should be fluctuated.

It is essential to note that if you are working with an athlete that you haven't had from a young age, the stage length does not have to be exactly as suggested above, where the ages are given in brackets. It is up to the coach to determine when the athlete should move into the next phase. Moreover, players develop at a vast range of different rates: the age ranges are given merely as a guide.

The table provides recommendations within each phase of strength development; it provides a guideline based on my experience and scientific research (see for example Baechle and Earle, 2000; Siff, 2003). Certain variables must be adjusted for individuals, taking into account other forms of training load they are undertaking. For example, you may have a scheduled work capacity phase and session to do with a particular athlete or team. An aspect to consider within this framework is the differences between certain athletes, as some will be able to tolerate more load than others. Although we need to hit a certain threshold for adaptation, that threshold will depend on each athlete individually. Identifying this threshold is an important skill in its own right for a coach/practitioner to develop, to know your athlete well and what should be prescribed for them in order to get the balance right for getting your athletes stronger and more robust, but not acutely causing them to break down. The idea is to apply the minimal dose possible for adaptation, although over reaching techniques are required at times. Again, this depends upon a particular athlete's genetic make-up and potential, in what is known in the scientific research as being a responder or non-responder to various stimuli

Strength development phase	Recommended sets	Recommended repetitions	Recommended recovery time
Fundamental movement patterns	Incorporate in games or warm-up drills	8–12	n/a
Motor control/intro	2–4	6–12	30–90 seconds
Work capacity/high volume strength	2–5	6–10 (sub-maximal level)	15–45 seconds
Increasing maximal strength	3–6	2–5 (progressing to maximal lifts) 6–8 (functional hypertrophy)	2–4 minutes

(Davidsen *et al.*, 2011). Unfortunately, the genetic make-up of athletes is out of anyone's control, so it is once again up to the coach to ensure that maximum adaptation can be made with their athletes. Another thing to consider is the workload and schedule the athletes are going through beyond the strength and conditioning (S&C) programme. It may be that the S&C does not cause any injury concerns, but the overall load may contribute to overload injuries.

Note that there is an extra repetition range in the strength section for functional hypertrophy, which could be used in certain aspects of the season or cycle. (Functional hypertrophy means there is an increase in muscle cross-sectional area that relates to a direct increase in force production.) My recommendation is that repetition range should never exceed this in a functional hypertrophy phase, otherwise the intensity and percentage of maximal load will have to decrease too much, eliciting a decrease in force production. It would also cause an increase in hypertrophy that is not functional, therefore producing size that would inhibit performance. In the earlier stages of strength development when motor control/work capacity is being performed, coaches do not need to worry about any unwanted hypertrophy as athletes are still learning motor skills and greater repetitions are potentially required (Stafford, 2005). However, there is definitely scope to prescribe higher repetition ranges to an athlete within an anatomical adaptation phase, or when the athlete is new to strength training. If done correctly it can also be implemented as a variation within a strength cycle to provide a two-week shock for the athlete and reduce the neurological stress. It can also complement a corrective exercise type programme, where a particular dysfunction is being fixed and then patterned into an integrated movement.

VOLUME VS. INTENSITY

There is a real debate in S&C literature and amongst practising coaches about whether a programme that is high-volume, high-intensity, or somewhere in between is the ideal prescription for optimal strength development; much depends on the coach's personal philosophy and experience within the field. There is no doubt that the fluctuation of training load is imperative not only for strength adaptation but for recovery (Stone *et al.*, 1999a; 1999b), although this periodized tool will be discussed in greater detail later on this textbook.

Furthermore, much depends on the type of sport, athlete and perception of high intensity/volume programmes. For example, there may be a need for greater strength volume throughout the week if strength is a greater priority in your sport. For example, a rugby player will have a number of consecutive sessions based on strength throughout the week; other team invasion sports such as football or hockey, although benefiting greatly from strength sessions, need to develop other physical qualities, so a lower volume of weekly and total strength work will therefore occur for these sports.

This book is not designed to specify how many strength sessions should be included in a particular sport or cycle phase, but instead to give careful consideration to the notion that there is more than one way of constructing and performing a well-implemented strength programme. The key exercises that follow provide an important stimulus for certain musculature and connective structures, and are necessary to optimize force production, essential for increasing strength and therefore reducing the potential for injury. Some of these exercises will be discussed in depth; others will be dealt with in general terms or listed within a key category.

Please note that although the exercises are prescribed with good scientific rationale, there will be cases where some athletes may not benefit from certain exercises at particular times, for example in a busy competition period or if an individual needs to fix dysfunctions prior to a strength programme. However, the exercises given below are recommended as tools for the majority of athletes.

······························

THE EXERCISES

The squat

Squatting is a well-known and documented exercise used in movement competencies and strength programmes. When performed correctly it can enhance an athlete's ability to triple extend (extension at the ankle, knee and hip) the lower limb under high force conditions (remember that force = mass × acceleration).

There is some disagreement amongst coaches as to how wide the stance should be. From experience, if an athlete struggles to get good depth, a wider stance can be adopted, although some tests such as the Functional Movement Screen (FMS) prohibit any stance wider than shoulder width to highlight any compensation (Cook, Burton and Hoogenboom, 2006) – in other words, if an athlete has to adopt a wider stance to get good depth in a squat, is the athlete compensating somewhere? For example, a lack of dorsiflexion within an athlete limits good depth so a wider stance would compensate and create the depth required. The coach then has to ensure that this dysfunction is addressed along with squatting work.

It is commonly believed that squats in general are bad for the knee joint, and that coaches should prevent athletes from allowing their knees to go over their toes. Although as coaches we should try to enforce the posterior tilt of the pelvis so the weight distribution goes through the heels, ensuring a greater activation of the posterior chain, there is no scientific evidence to support that knees going over the toes is detrimental to knee health. In fact, contrasting research demonstrates that squatting does not exert high forces on the knee, or place the anterior cruciate ligament (ACL) under much strain (Escamilla, 2001). In fact, greater dorsiflexion ability within the squat would enable better movement and less compensation at other joints so ensuring the knees go over the toes as much as possible will enhance ankle mobility.

What is very well-known and conclusive, however, is the depth required when performing the squat exercise. If an athlete reaches a depth of the legs where they are parallel to the floor or deeper, there is a greater shift of activation to the gluteus groups of muscles (Caterisano et al., 2002), also known as the posterior chain of the lower limb, but not so much for the hamstrings (Isear, Erickson and Worrel, 1997). Since more or less all of the sports are quadriceps-dominant, due to the repetitive smaller ranges of movement of the hip and knee joint required to perform the sporting activities, it is essential that this exercise elicits a greater stimulus to the posterior chain in an attempt to balance the strength levels in the lower limb. Alongside deep squatting exercises, athletes need to be performing specific hamstring exercises; these will be discussed further in the next section. As briefly discussed in the introduction to strength training, note that for a reduction in knee injuries, the posterior chain in particular should be strengthened for greater control and stability at the hip and knee joints.

Significant performance benefits can be gained with squats that are partial in depth, as the specificity of force production is greater than sporting movement itself. However, with partial squatting, the dominant muscles required for the movement are the quadriceps, which counteract the balancing operation of the lower limb. There is rationale at certain

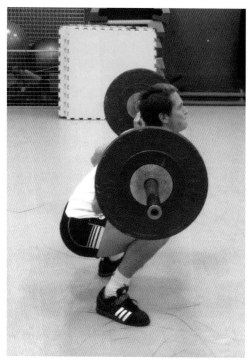 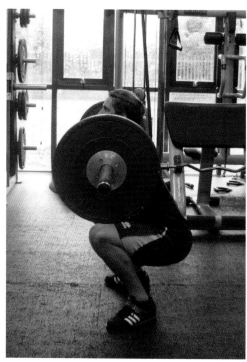

Back and front squat exercises, with full ROM for enhancing triple extension strength of the lower limb.

phases of the cycle/season, however, for implementing high force partial squats, as the load being lifted would be significantly greater, causing neurological overload, as there will be an optimal length tension relation for generating high levels of force (Hill, 1953; Huxley, 1957). The majority of the training prescription should be reinforcing good depth of a squat, from an injury prevention point of view. As mentioned above, the gluteus group of muscles can be targeted within deep squatting exercises; the coach also needs to elicit techniques that strengthen the hamstring group of muscles for an effective injury prevention programme.

Although for a healthy athlete with good mobility the squat exercise is an extremely effective exercise to use, it must be noted that it isn't always the best exercise to use with some athletes. For example, if an athlete has poor ankle mobility, then they will search for more depth with compensation at other joints. Therefore, squatting may not be in their programme and enhancing ankle mobility will be an emphasis within their prehab programmes. With this athlete then, the leg press may be used as an alternative to a squat exercise. This will be more thoroughly discussed in the Chapter 3, and demonstrated in the applied case study; however, coaches need to provide individualized programmes.

Eccentric loading exercises

The eccentric phase of an exercise is often known as the negative or downward phase, and there are many exercises that focus on this eccentric part in particular for strengthening. It must be stated, firstly, that eccentric training focuses on applying tension to a muscle while it lengthens as opposed to when it shortens in the concentric phase. For the hamstrings in particular, exercises such as the Romanian deadlift (RDL), good morning, and Nordic exercise are examples of eccentrically loading the hamstrings. Exercises such as the RDL will enhance the hamstring strength whilst hinging from the hip when the knee joint is close to extension. The Nordic exercise is completed whilst the knee joint is flexed, so the two exercises should be completed together within a hamstring programme. Eccentric loading exercises provide a direct stimulus to improve the strength of these muscles as they are said to have greater strength responses than concentric training alone (Roig *et al.*, 2009), and reduce injury rates within athletes (Croisier *et al.*, 2008: Olsen *et al.*, 2005). Exercises such as the Nordic hamstring exercise can be implemented with very young and novice athletes; providing athletes can control their own bodyweight under eccentric load, they will be a thorough starting point for the progression of eccentric loading. In my experience, exercises that concentrically activate the hamstrings, such as leg curls, should be avoided, as lengthening the hamstrings is essential for injury prevention. Eccentric training can also be applied to all exercises as the lengthening/downward phase can be emphasized. A spotter is required, though, as the athlete should be able to eccentrically control up to approximately 120 per cent of their concentric one repetition max (1RM) (Roig *et al.*, 2009), with assistance on the concentric phase to lift the load. This eccentric high load method can be utilized with many strength exercises, not just hamstring-conditioning ones.

Isometric hamstring conditioning

Although eccentric hamstring training has been endorsed and encouraged in most recent years for reducing hamstring injuries, there is a small argument against it. When hamstring injuries occur generally, it does so when the hamstrings are in a brief isometric state close to full extension of the knee joint. Therefore, the practitioner is encouraged to incorporate some isometric conditioning of the hamstrings within their injury prevention programmes. Exercise such as back hyperextensions and bridges with the legs close to full extension would be examples of this.

High intensity running

As well as looking at enhancing the eccentric loading of the hamstring group of muscles, it is important that they are conditioned under higher velocity actions as well. Within many sports, the amount of maximal sprints that occurs over 30m is limited within technical/tactical training and the majority of game play. Therefore, the hamstrings are generally unconditioned over longer distances when fatigue starts to occur. It is therefore imperative that some longer distance sprinting, or close to sprinting, is placed within an athlete's programme so they are exposed to this type of repetitive hamstring contraction. The hamstrings have to load eccentrically at a rapid rate when at the end of extension, whereas resistance exercises such as the RDL and Nordic only provide a slower eccentric contraction. The coach can build up the distance/repetitions/sets when they feel it is appropriate for that athlete/sport. Furthermore, it is essential that athletes are exposed to this type of stimuli for a reduced risk of hamstring injury.

High force producing exercises: Focus on the 'deadlift'

As mentioned briefly earlier in this text, maximizing an athlete's force-producing capabilities will increase the robustness and integrity of that area. Therefore, another important injury prevention tool will dedicate time to maximizing force-producing capabilities. The partial squat, which has been mentioned previously in the context of maximizing force capabilities, should be used sparingly throughout a periodized programme. However, an exercise such as the deadlift, where the bar must be lifted from the ground with good posture, can generate greater load/weight. Remember that force is equal to mass × acceleration, so lifting the most mass with the greatest speed or intention

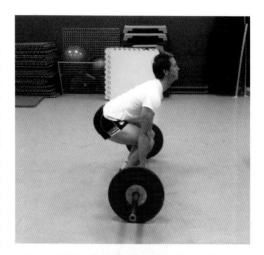

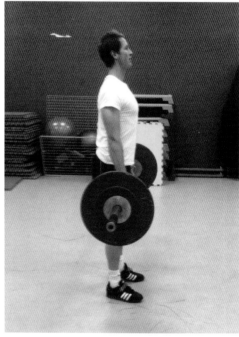

Starting and finishing positions of the deadlift exercise. It is important to maintain this posture over the bar throughout the lift. Stand fully erect to complete the lift.

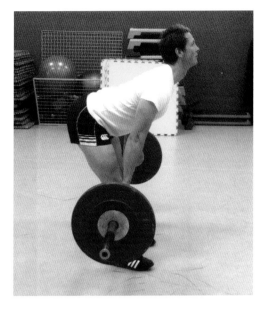

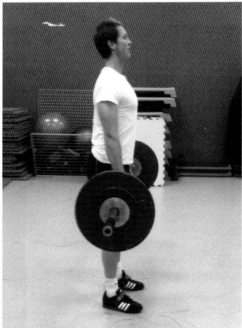

Starting and finishing positions for the Romanian deadlift exercise. Move the bottom back as far as possible, whilst the bar travels down the front of the legs. Keep legs as straight as possible to load the hamstrings more. As usual, posture is key: maintain the neutral spine position throughout.

to lift fast will ensure greater force production and strength adaptation. Further, it is important to understand that maximizing force is only a part of an injury prevention programme and other modalities are essential. If attempting to maximize the force and load lifted in this exercise, the use of straps must be permitted in order to avoid a weak grip limiting force producing capabilities in the triple extension position.

Olympic lifts such as the clean-and-jerk and snatch are common weightlifting exercises used in the field of strength and conditioning. Though they provide some injury prevention benefit, they are designed to increase explosive strength and power, and therefore are used more as a performance enhancement tool. These lifts will therefore not be discussed at length within this textbook.

Upper body strength exercises

A common issue amongst certain athletes when training the upper body is an obsession with wanting to do exercises that enhance aesthetic qualities of their physique, not performance qualities. Although these 'non-functional' exercises (the bicep curl and chest fly, for example) could be placed in a particular athlete's programme at some point, with good justification and rationale, it is essential that athletes are reminded that going to the gym and just performing this type of exercise will not enhance their performance. Instead, upper body exercises should be compound lifts: a push/pull in both horizontal and vertical planes. Horizontal force production includes key exercises such as the bench press and bent-over row/bench row, whilst vertical force production lifts include shoulder/push press and pull-ups. Although there are many exercises that could be implemented, these are the main four types of lift, essential for a strength programme focused around the upper body.

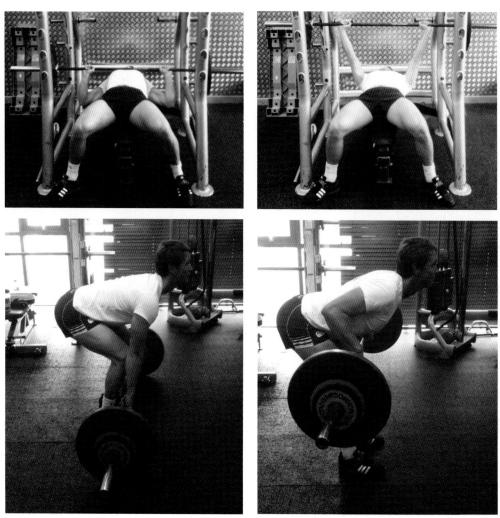

These exercises demonstrate the technical aspects of the two horizontal push/pull complexes – the bench press and the bent over row. It is important in the bench press that the athlete pushes through the ground to generate force and extend the arms as fast as possible. The bent over row exercise ensures the athlete gets the upper body as parallel to the floor as possible, promoting effective hinging patterns also.

There is much debate amongst practitioners within the field of strength and conditioning about which force direction application (vertical or horizontal) is more beneficial in the transference of strength to the sporting arena. This debate is often based on coaches' personal opinion without scientific evidence, although provides an insight to real day-to-day work in the strength and conditioning field. Many coaches believe that vertical pushing, for example, including shoulder press exercises, are best for transference to the sporting arena, as they have greater similarities to the extension of the elbow and shoulder joints in many sporting actions (such as a punch, throw, or hand-off in rugby). On the other hand, many coaches feel that trying to specify and copy the direction of force application defeats the object of maximizing force-producing capabilities. Furthermore, the bench press exercise, a horizontal pressing exercise, elicits greater force production than a vertical press such as the shoulder press, as the amount of load lifted can be maximized. (The force equation ($F=ma$) ought to be in the forefront of a strength and conditioning coach's mind.) As with the lower limb, increasing the strength of the upper limb musculature and connective structures will

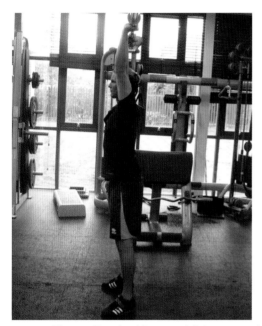
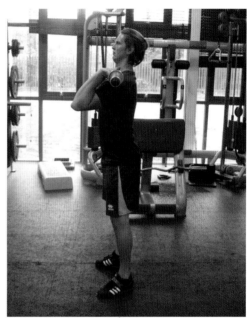

The standing shoulder press. It is important that the athlete can maintain erect posture and transfer force efficiently.

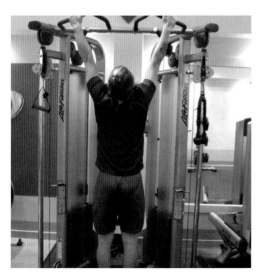
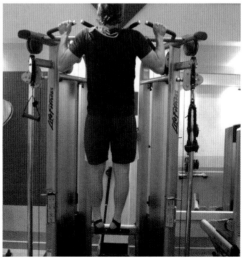

The pull-up exercise.

significantly reduce injuries, due to the higher forces the limb will be able to tolerate. Ensuring that force production is high and a compound lift is performed, the exercise must be bilateral (i.e. lifting with two limbs), as this produces the greatest load lifted and force. There is, however, a place for unilateral strength training; this will discussed in much greater detail in the next section.

Bilateral vs. unilateral force production

It has already been well documented that bilateral strength training is essential for maximizing force production and creating the optimal stimulus for strength development, which has been proven successful in injury reduction. However, a strength programme

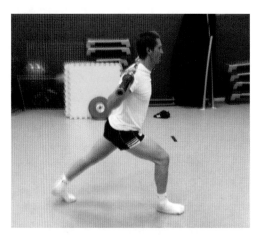
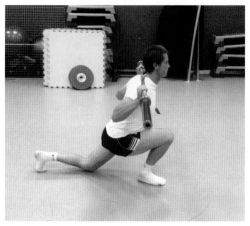
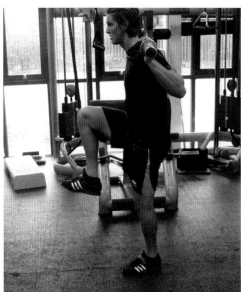
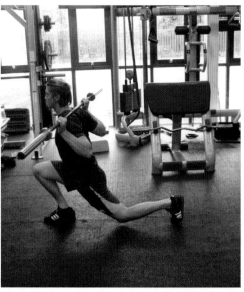

The exercise above demonstrates both the split squat (top) and lunge (bottom) exercise. The split squat seems the logical starting point with unilateral exercises before prescribing lunging exercises, as there is a natural progression from more static to dynamic unilateral exercises. Notice the finishing position where greater dorsiflexion is promoted whilst still pushing through the heels.

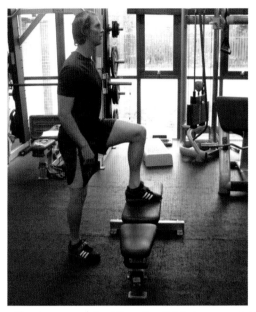 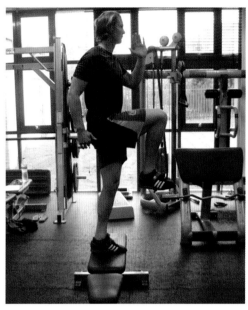

The step-up exercise. When the athlete becomes stable enough, the height of the step can be increased to ensure the unilateral strength can be generated through full ROM.

should include unilateral work (i.e. placing stress to each limb under isolation within an exercise), as this bridges the gap between bilateral force production and the sum of unilateral force production (Behm and Andersen, 2006). For example, an athlete could focus on the symmetry between each limb and test if one leg/arm is significantly stronger than the other. In certain sports it might be an accepted aim to have one leg physically stronger, as that limb will require greater work/load in competition – therefore trying to reach a complete balance and homeostatic state within the two limbs could actually reduce time spent on maximizing the physical performance and robustness of the 'strong' limb. For example, the dominant racket hand in any racket sport would ideally be the stronger limb to tolerate the high load and forces they have to go through. In many other sports, and potentially the majority of sports, the weaker limb needs to be as close as possible in strength terms to the stronger limb.

This is essential to avoid any deficits in movement and avoiding any limb over-compensating as this could lead to potential injuries. In particular, increasing the stability of the limb under isolation is essential for the knee and would provide a significantly more stable limb. This technique, although not optimal for maximal strength development, provides a good foundation for each limb (Behm and Andersen, 2006). Examples of key exercises that are unilateral for the lower limb would include lunges, step-ups, and Hungarian split squats.

Examples of unilateral exercises for the upper limb would be any type of dumbbell pressing in either a horizontal and vertical direction of force production, or a dumbbell row, best performed in a horizontal position. Eccentrically loading the hamstrings for an effective injury prevention tool, mentioned earlier, is implemented with unilateral exercises. Exercises such as single leg RDLs and arabesque-type movements can look at eccentrically loading the hamstrings on one limb, assessing the ability to hip hinge and avoid rotation of the hips to achieve the greatest hip flexion possible. These types of points and movement exercises will also be discussed in greater detail in the movement preparation section in Chapter 8 (Maturing and Youth Athletes). It is important to note (this is not discussed in textbooks but is more derived from personal experience) that with unilateral exercises a little higher volume is required for greatest strength and stability gains. Therefore, intensity will be lower (in the sense of lifting a lower percentage of 1RM), but more repetitions should be performed. For example, if three repetitions are being performed in the high force exercises, then a recommended five repetitions should be performed on each limb in the unilateral exercises.

To summarize the focus on bilateral and unilateral strength training: bilateral strength training requires exercises to be executed with two limbs and the greatest amount of load lifted. Unilateral exercises are performed on one leg at a time, and therefore require each limb to be placed under tension in isolation, and increase the stability of the joints of the limb.

As well as enhancing the force production within unilateral exercises, these types of exercises offer an important stimulus for injury prevention. Ensuring good control on single limb exercises can be managed, which requires the athlete to show great single limb stability, with good control of the joints and stabilizers that ensure the movement occurs. For example, a single leg squatting pattern requires good stabilization of the knee to ensure the movement is performed correctly. Perform the exercise with lower load and focus on the eccentric phase of the exercise, and in particular on the movement of the knee joint. This type of single leg stability work should be an integral part of the injury prevention programme and could be included in warm-up sets prior to bilateral and unilateral higher force work. Single leg stability work will be discussed in greater detail later, and the importance of this work must be recognized in relation to higher force strength training.

EXERCISE ORDER: PUTTING THE STRENGTH PROGRAMME TOGETHER

Before progressing onto other modalities related to strength training and injury prevention, it is essential to now piece together an effective injury prevention strength programme, and outline correct order sequence to maximize adaptation. The session as a whole might focus not only on maximal strength but power and velocity aspects also, as it could be a combination of injury prevention and performance enhancement within the weights room; the two generally go well together. If any plyometric work, Olympic lifting and so on is prescribed, this should be prioritized at the start of the programme, before the maximal/general strength work. Then the strength work begins and it is important to follow the flow chart below, so that exercises are completed with maximal effort and therefore maximal adaptation occurs. From a strength perspective, as evident in the graph below, you can see all the lower limb exercises go first: bilateral and then unilateral. This is because the lower limb would be more taxing physiologically/neurologically, and is generally the most important aspect of athletic performance. Then the upper body proceeds, where the muscle recruitment is lower and is less neurologically taxing and so on. Within each region of the body, it is essential that bilateral exercises always come first as you are trying to maximize force production when the athlete is fresher. The unilateral exercises are known as supplementary exercises. Any prehab modality that has not been discussed in this book will be performed before any of the lifting as part of the warm up. If a programme consists of a lot of necessary prehab exercises, then it can be incorporated in between lifting sets. (These modalities will be discussed in detail throughout this book.) There is a much debate within the field about at what point trunk stability work is performed. Many believe it should be performed at the end of the session; I find it useful to place it within the prehab section at the start, depending of course on the intensity/volume of work.

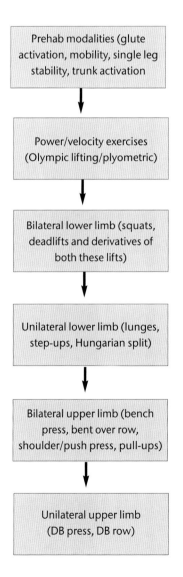

GLUTEAL/POSTERIOR CHAIN ACTIVATION

The importance of the posterior chain in preventing injuries has already been discussed, with particular focus on hamstring strength and how to increase this through specific eccentric loading exercises. Another important anatomical region of the posterior chain that hasn't been discussed is the gluteals, which get greater activation in deep squats than the hamstrings or quadriceps (Caterisano et al., 2002). This section will focus on other prehab modalities to increase the activity of gluteal muscles and how to increase their functionality. In general the glutes are a stabilizing muscle that can enhance the efficiency of movement and provide power and strength within explosive performance. From an injury prevention perspective, the gluteus maximus, the largest and more superficial muscle in the glutes, can be significantly activated in exercises that cause full ROM in hip flexion/extension. For example, deep squatting is essential for glute activation and strengthening to assist the hamstring development, as discussed earlier. The importance of exercises such as the deep squat for posterior chain development and injury prevention is now becoming apparent. Any unilateral exercise of the lower limb, such as the lunge, has greater gluteal activation than bilateral exercises alone (Bodreau et al., 2005). Unilateral exercises also demonstrate greater activation of another glute muscle, the gluteus medius, and is primarily responsible for any hip abduction. 'Glute med', although worked globally in unilateral lower limb strength exercises, can be isolated in exercises prior to training in an attempt to activate them and act as an effective injury prevention tool. Weak gluteus medius can lead to issues regarding the knee also, in particular causing knee valgus, i.e. the inward rotation of the knee. Working on the gluteus medius in conjunction with the other global posterior chain movements can potentially rectify this, and ensure the knee is more stable; creating greater stability with the knee is essential for greater health and function of the knee in particular. On the other hand, although it is essential that the hip abductors are strong, glute medius may play only a small role. There are other smaller hip abductor muscles that could be as important to strengthening the hip abductors. However, if done correctly, all the exercises shown should enhance hip abduction strength in general, including all relevant musculature. Please see below exercises that can be performed within a glute activation session; the session takes 10 minutes and should be carried out prior to any physical session or even technical/tactical training –due to its short length this is usually possible.

EXERCISE TECHNICAL DESCRIPTION

Glute bridge

Lie on the ground with legs bent at 90 degrees and feet firmly on the ground. Raise pelvis off the ground so hips are fully extended and get athlete to squeeze in their glutes. Get the athletes to 'peel' off the ground to ensure effective pelvic movement, and push through the heels.

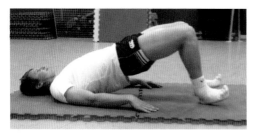

Straight leg glute bridge

Same technique as a normal glute bridge, but one leg is put straight and raised off the ground so one limb is isolated. Ensure the

pelvis is stable when performing the exercise.

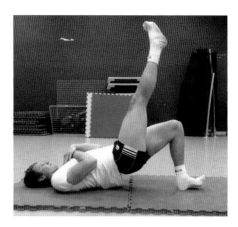

Hip abductor

Performed sitting or standing, ensure body is erect and in a straight line and raise the leg out to the side, keeping it straight. Perform with internal rotation of the foot to activate glute medius further.

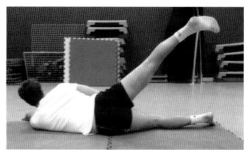

Clamshell

Lie on the ground on your side with legs bent, and abduct your leg in the flexed position. This should only be used with novice athletes for the first few weeks of their programme. After

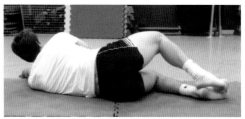

this, this exercise does not elicit enough adaptation.

Lateral band walks

In a partial squat position, move laterally, keeping feet a constant width apart as the band places tension on the glute med.

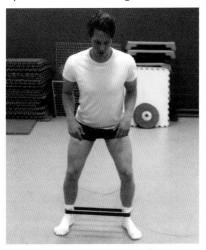

Monster walks

With the band, walk in a diagonal pattern abducting the leg at every step. Can be performed backwards as well.

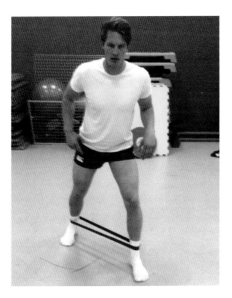

Band squats

With tension on the band around the knees, get your athlete to squat as deep as they can with extra tension on the hip abductors. Encourage the athlete to pull the knees apart when performing the squat.

Progress this to single leg squats with the band still in position.

It is essential, however, that even with the glute activation exercises that they are progressed to apply a greater stimulus for adaptation, known as overload. This is a key philosophy within any training modality, where the athlete doesn't get exposed to the same stimulus over and over again. In this scenario, the glute bridge can be progressed by adding load across the hips with a bar (see picture). Of course, more volume can be added but eventually intensity should be increased. There are obviously times within a programme where intensity and volume will be reduced, as fluctuation of load is essential for the recovery of an athlete (Stone *et al.*, 1999a, 1999b), which will be discussed in greater detail in the next chapter. However, for the maximal adaptation of a physical quality, overload, however it is achieved, is essential. It is essential to know that this method and the exercises shown in the table above are an acute activation of the posterior chain and therefore a direct attempt to prevent injuries

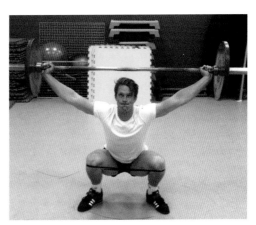

and enhance performance.

With posterior chain activation exercises, in an attempt to activate the gluteal muscles, there must be a continuum coaches follow. For example, apart from the last exercise provided in the table above, the exercises are known as isolation exercises of the glutes, and in isolation will activate the required glute muscle at low thresholds. The last example (band squats) provides an example of an integration exercise of the posterior chain. This is where the movement becomes more dynamic and as a coach, you're asking the athlete to now recruit the posterior chain muscles within a particular motor pattern. Coaches should ensure that they do not leave this aspect out, and that there is an isolation exercise or group of exercises that follow into an integration exercise. Other exercises that would integrate the glutes are lunges, single leg squats and their derivatives (bilateral squatting, etc.). The coach must ensure firstly that the athlete has the ability to activate their glutes during these integrated exercises. If the athlete does not have an ability to do this, they should focus on the isolation exercises initially. Although the posterior chain is essential within athletes' well-being and injury prevention programmes, each individual athlete needs to be assessed separately, as one training method may not be applicable for all. In my experience, some athletes as well as not having great posterior chain strength, have poor muscular strength and size within the vastus medialis oblique (VMO). This has led to poor tracking of the knee and further issues when loading higher volumes of sporting movements. In this case, it would be recommended that some leg extension, focusing on the end range of extension be prescribed to activate and stimulate VMO for increased strength and hypertrophy. The coach and practitioner therefore need to know their athletes and assess them appropriately before any core lifts and supplementary strength exercises are prescribed. In some cases, traditional S&C lifts aren't always appropriate in isolation and a coach needs to have an open mind towards other techniques appropriate for certain athletes.

OTHER CONSIDERATIONS

It is impossible to over-estimate the importance of maximal strength, from a strength and conditioning coach's point of view, and it should always remain a part of an athlete's physical programme. However, the S&C coach needs to consider the benefits of the whole programme around the strength work. Within busy periods of competition, or if physical emphasis shifts to another aspect in training, strength prescription needs to be considered. The coach cannot prescribe high volumes of maximal strength work all year round irrespective of what the athlete is doing within their sporting training. At times, strength training needs to be reduced and focus should be placed on other aspects of the athlete's development. It must also be recognized that some athletes cannot handle high volumes of strength work on top of their training load within their sports. This could be due to a dysfunction causing the athlete to compensate elsewhere, leading to overload of a certain anatomical region. The coach needs to highlight those athletes susceptible to overload injuries and ensure the total load is not too high, and their dysfunction is fixed. Therefore, the coach should consider the minimal dose response that an athlete would need for adaptation to avoid any negative outcome.

2 | MANAGING RECOVERY AND AVOIDING OVERTRAINING

As well as reducing injury potential from an acute perspective, longitudinal and chronic injuries that are experienced over time must be avoided, and it is the role of the strength and conditioning coach to ensure this happens. There are many techniques available in the field to enhance recovery and avoid overtraining. (Note, however, that the term 'overtraining' is now technically incorrect and should be termed 'unexplained underperformance syndrome' (UPS).) UPS consists of there either being a plateau or decrease in performance, even when a well-designed overloaded training programme is still in place (Budgett, 2000). There are many physiological markers that can be associated with an overtrained state, which this book will not cover; readers particularly interested in this aspect are directed to the References section. It is more noticeable and common in endurance athletes due to a significantly higher volume of physiological load. Although this chapter will focus on avoiding UPS it will also emphasize the importance of reducing general fatigue and maximizing recovery. Aside from the various recovery tools available, which are discussed in greater detail in the latter part of this chapter, it is essential that the focus is on periodization, and planning effective recovery times within micro-, meso- and macro-cycles to ensure that effective rest and maximum adaptation occur. It is often forgotten that when designing a periodized programme for enhancing any physical quality, the best recovery tool is a well-designed programme with sufficient recovery time integrated (Haff, 2004a, 2004b). Remember, fatigue is a product of not enough recovery time, not too much of a training stimulus, although the two often correlate strongly (Budgett, 2000).

PERIODIZATION

There are many definitions for the term, but in its simplest form 'periodization' means an effectively planned programme with clear emphasis on particular qualities and clear indication of the fluctuation of volume and intensity of work (Siff, 2003). Variables associated with volume and intensity will be discussed in greater detail in this section of the chapter; choosing the correct variables will depend on the sport, the athlete, the experience of the athlete/coach and the resources available. Furthermore, there will be a discussion on quantifying both volume and intensity within physiological/mechanical loads, in an attempt to plan, monitor and prescribe a programme that generates progress and overload for adaptation, and manages fatigue for a potential injury reduction.

VOLUME

'Volume' is defined as the amount of work done in a particular session/cycle, hence the accumulated loading that has been placed on the athlete (Plisk and Stone, 2003). This section will outline simple ways volume can be calculated or quantified, either with simple, inexpensive methods or with greater technology where the level of detail can increase. It must be stressed, however, that a thorough job can be performed with methods that are cost-free. When calculating volume, it is essential that consideration is made to both physiological and mechanical load. Mechanical load is what we will focus on firstly; specifically looking at how we calculate volume in the gym/weights room and the physiological load in the sporting environment following that.

There are many techniques and methods available for assessing mechanical load, the first being a simple form of calculating the total number of repetitions performed. This would provide a simple idea of whether it was a high- or low-volume session. It must be noted that the comparison of repetitions are only relative to each team or individual player; comparisons between one player and another and between different teams should be avoided. There is no number that represents a high or low volume: it will purely depend on the athlete's tolerance, and coach's philosophy as to what a high-volume session is.

Another, more accurate, method for potentially calculating volume is to calculate volume load (Haff, 2010):

Volume load = number of repetitions × number of sets × load lifted

Volume load is then collected for every exercise performed and then added together to get a total session volume load. It is important once again that the load number is only used as a planning/comparison tool within one team/player. It should not be compared to other teams as it will become inaccurate due to many other variables. Remember also that volume load can only be compared against sessions with the same content, for example with the same exercises. This is because load lifted is incorporated within the equation for calculating volume load. As we are aware, the amount of weight lifted fluctuates with varying exercises, as it depends on what musculature is responsible for lifting the load. For example, a deadlift would require greater musculature than the bench press exercise and would therefore provide greater load lifted. Therefore, direct volume load comparison between the deadlift exercise and the bench press cannot occur. If a comparison is to be made between sessions that are different in content, it would be more scientifically precise to compare volume using total repetitions. Even though volume load provides a more advanced tool to calculate volume, it is not always more precise and the practitioner should select carefully the one to be used.

Physiological volume can potentially be more difficult to quantify, especially as the sport could dictate how it is approached. In its simplest form with any modality or sport, total minutes that athletes spend on their feet can be used. There is an obvious flaw with this method: an athlete can 'train' for a period of time but the time does not indicate what happened within it. It does, however, if you know your athlete and how they are working, provide an indicator of the volume of a session. A more advanced method of calculating physiological volume is assessing distance covered. This is easier within both strict physiological sports such as endurance events, and with speed events because the distance of the interval or training session is usually known or easier to calculate. However, within a team sport where the play and game itself dictates the movement of the athlete some advanced technology is required. The most commonly used technology in professional sport is Global Positioning System (GPS), which can assess the distance covered within a selected period of time. This software can also give us a breakdown of how the distance is covered; for example, it will set a threshold of speeds, and if an athlete goes over that certain threshold, it will be classified as a particular category. For example, there is a high intensity running speed category (and slower speed categories prior to that). The high speed running zone set within the GPS system I have had experience with is 19.8–24.4 km/h (STAT Sport). Anything above 24.4km/h is therefore classed as a maximal sprint. The issue for me, when speeds are already preset for certain thresholds, is that you neglect a huge proportion of individualized monitoring. These thresholds should (in an ideal world) be set for each individual based on a percentage of peak velocity, not a set speed for everyone. An example of good practice can be found in a study by Buchheit *et al.* (2010), in which maximal velocity data was obtained, and percentages of speed from each individual player were calculated. Martin Buchheit adjusted the high speed running zone to 61 per cent of every athlete's maximal velocity. Although Buchheit's percentage is arbitrary, and it is unclear why this figure was selected, the standardized parameters set by the current

Total Distance Covered	100 km	Volume calculation	Volume of speed
10–11km/h	10	10.5 × 10	105
11–12km/h	20	11.5 × 20	230
12–13km/h	10	12.5 × 10	125
13–14km/h	5	13.5 × 5	67.5
14–15km/h	5	14.5 × 5	72.5
15–16km/h	5	15.5 × 5	77.5
16–17km/h	45	16.5 × 45	742.5
1425 Total volume			

Example of Player A within a training session.

Total Distance Covered	100km	Volume calculation	Volume of speed
10–11km/h	20	10.5 × 20	210
11–12km/h	25	11.5 × 25	287.5
12–13km/h	20	12.5 × 20	250
13–14km/h	15	13.5 × 15	202.5
14–15km/h	10	14.5 × 10	145
15–16km/h	5	15.5 × 5	77.5
16–17km/h	5	16.5 × 5	82.5
			1255 Total Volume

Example of Player B within a training session.

software companies provide limited monitoring. You can be creative in calculating a really accurate volume load using GPS, which can incorporate volume and intensity. If you multiply the distance covered by the amount of time that was spent at that speed, you can create an extremely accurate volume, which can differentiate between volumes that have spent more time at higher speeds. The examples in the tables give the total volume for two separate players, A and B.

The examples, although potentially inaccurate in terms of actual speeds as the ranges either side can be stretched further within team sports, still demonstrate the difference in volume when taking into consideration the speeds at which athletes move within the distance covered. The formula used was very simple: it took the average number between each speed category, and multiplied that by how much distance was covered within that speed. It was then added together to give a total volume. The speeds covered should be normalized; for example, player A may have a maximal speed of 24km/h, whereas player B has 22km/h. Therefore, it will be easier for player A to hit greater distances at higher speeds as it is a relatively lower percentage, so results could be misleading. Within intensity quantification, therefore, it is important that relative thresholds are used, if possible, to ensure the intensities of individuals can be comparable to the whole group, as reinforced by Dr Martin Buchheit's 2010 study.

Other key variables that require serious consideration include high metabolic load (HML), which is derived from an algorithm and formula preset by the software company – this is considered the gold standard measuring variable. HML takes into account all the variables although is very heavily influenced by distance covered. Others that are essential are acceleration and deceleration, calculated at the speed of increase/decrease of starting/stopping. These key factors should be monitored in conjunction with other variables and may depict a different type of session and stress placed on the body. Therefore, certain variables can be targeted to overload certain physiological qualities. As an example, a high number of acceleration/decelerations would be an indicator of a more anaerobic session, with increasing of buffering qualities of acidosis and potentially repeated sprint ability. On the other side, higher HML or total distance covered would indicate a session more focused on aerobic development. If the coach wants to periodize the technical/tactical physiological load on field, they can overload certain variables from the GPS data, and provide a saturated stimulus for a certain physiological quality.

INTENSITY

Whereas volume is defined as the quantity of work, intensity is defined as the quality of work. Although low intensity is not always poor in quality, it is fair to say a high intensity session would be closer to maximal (Chadd, 2010). Quantifying mechanical intensity within the gym provides a method that many strength and conditioning coaches know, but very rarely apply. Athletes that have had a good training history within resistance training would use percentage of their one repetition maximum (1RM) as a measure. Extensive data and guidelines are available to suggest what percentage should be used to elicit certain goals; for example, any strength adaptation must provide intensities of work at 85 per cent 1RM and above with well trained athletes (Tan, 1999); however, it is essential that every athlete doesn't follow the exact same percentage as some could see benefits with slightly lower percentages, especially if they are new to resistance training. Again, this reinforces the need for the coach to know particular athletes and adjust accordingly. Within this technique however, it is important to test players' 1RM regularly to ensure percentages of 1RM are correct for quantifying intensity. The testing of 1RM can often be done in training to save time, and be more practical. For example, the phase focus could be to maximize high force qualities, therefore some singles or one repetition will be completed during the training session. Many coaches, however, use an estimated 1RM which is provided or estimated via assessment of the athlete's training. Although not completely accurate scientifically, for those who know their athletes well, it will save time and still be a good indicator for training intensity. Examples of two different methods within two different population groups are by Comfort *et al.* (2014) and Harvat *et al.* (2003).

With athletes who are developing, or do not have a good training history, and therefore cannot test a 1RM, or wouldn't even be training in thresholds that high yet, it would be recommended that a scale of intensity is used. For example, as a coach you could have a scale as simple as 1–5, 1 being the lowest and 5 being the highest. You would assign a number for each player and each session to provide a quantification of the intensity levels within the gym, or even within physiological intensity (to be discussed shortly). The coach can classify the session from an intensity point of view; however, it must be remembered that this is not a classification of physiological intensity, but a classification of mechanical load and neurological stress. Further, if a session elicits low load in terms of weight but includes a high heart-rate stimulus, like a circuit type session, it should be classified as a low mechanical intensity session. These scores/scales issued from the coach can also be combined with an athlete Rating of Perceived Exertion (RPE), commonly known as the Borg Scale. If used correctly, although criticized for being too subjective and dependent on emotional factors during the session (Dunbar *et al.*, 1992), it can add value and weight to the intensity of the session from an athlete's perspective. There must be a process of athlete education explaining the scale rating and what each number represents. From experience, RPE is best used with physiological loading rather than mechanical/neuromuscular because players' perceptions of maximal strength work with long recoveries provide low RPE scores; in turn the strength and conditioning specialist will understand the neuromuscular fatigue this session will inhibit, hence it needs to be recognized as a high mechanical intensity session. A recommendation that the modified Borg Scale from 1–10 is used, as opposed to the 6–20, as it is simpler and has been found more effective for athletes and their coaches (Turner *et al.*, 2014).

When quantifying physiological intensity there is much more emphasis on precision, perhaps since the majority of higher level clubs have the knowledge and equipment to execute it. First we will consider intensity from an intrinsic point of view, looking at percentage of heart rate (HR) max. There are recommendations on training zones for heart rates and although these can be conveyed in much greater detail, a basic outline will be shown below. It is important however, that practitioners obtain a maximal heart rate figure, or if that is not possible, then an estimated one is attained. The most used estimated HR max is simply 220 minus the athlete's age, although be aware that this comes with a degree of standard error, due to the variation amongst individuals with the same chronological age.

Although these percentages can be altered

Training zone	Per cent of HR max
Recovery	50–60
'Fat burning'	60–70
Aerobic training zone	70–80
Anaerobic threshold	80–90
Speed interval	90–100

This screenshot is taken from a particular athlete's programme that I have constructed. It demonstrates how volume load and intensity is calculated. Although it cannot be seen clearly (the screen shot was too large for the page), the intensity (per cent 1RM) is averaged for overall session intensity on the far right hand side of the template.

according to physiological responses and adaptations, they act as a guideline for intensity zones and physiological emphasis. The zones shown in the table act primarily as a tool of emphasis for more strict physiological sports, such as middle/long distance running, swimming, cycling, rowing, etc. In team sports, unless doing a prioritized one-to-one session regarding a particular physiological outcome, one training zone will not be targeted throughout a sports specific training session, and athletes will probably spend time in all of them. Therefore, values (such as peak and average values) are generally more useful in quantifying the physiological intensity of a session (Aubert, Seps and Beckers, 2003). In particular, the Aubert study proposed the training impulse (TRIMP) method of calculating training load, by calculating average HR multiplied by session duration. TRIMP is essentially the area under the curve on a HR trace. For intermittent sports, the average heart rate could be a poor indicator of

the intensity stress within practice/games (Turner et al., 2014). Therefore, more detail has to be implemented within HR analysis that indicates time spent at high heart rate zones. It must be remembered also that the heart is a muscle, and needs sufficient recovery from stress to adapt.

Another measurement that can be taken if accessible, to assist with HR data, is lactate levels. Without delving too much into the details of physiology, lactate is a good indicator of the amount of acidosis and inorganic phosphates, in particular hydrogen ions in the blood (Coutts et al., 2009). There are also strong correlations between lactate, heart rate and perceived exertions. If blood lactates rise to 2mmol, which is known as the lactate threshold, and subsequently further to 4mmol, it is said to have hit the lactate turnpoint and anaerobic threshold, which means the blood is more acidic; the intensity will potentially be higher and so will fatigue (Kindermann, Simon and Keul, 1979). Training

Monday							
Gym			Field			Mon	
	Duration	RPE	Vol.	Duration	RPE	Vol	Daily Vol.
Player A	60	7	420	90	6	540	960
Player B	75	8	600	95	5	475	1075

This table demonstrates a daily monitoring tool of volume and intensity using duration of training and RPE to calculate training load. Although this tool has flaws physiologically, it nevertheless provides a quick and inexpensive way of calculating volume loads.

recommendations should not be based on lactate values alone, but should assist HR values and RPE scores, to give an overall picture of the intensity of a session. When conducting the initial physiological test for maximal HR and the lactate threshold test, it is important for the more strict physiological sports listed earlier, mainly endurance based, that speeds are assigned with those HR and lactate values so training thresholds are easily prescribed.

Another physiological method used to quantify intensities within training programmes would be percentage of VO2 max, which is essentially the maximum volume of O2 an individual can inhale and direct to the working muscles. This value may be completed in a maximal step test within a laboratory, where VO2 max, HR max and lactate threshold can be all determined within the same test, providing clear training recommendations for intensity levels and speeds.

Along with the intrinsic intensity measures such as HR and lactate, all the variables discussed with the GPS can provide an effective extrinsic output of intensity. The coach can then provide an internal workload for a selected external output which would give them a measure of how efficient that athlete is physiologically.

If a physiology lab is not accessible, and an aerobic training session is to be prescribed based on some testing result, a coach can use maximal aerobic speed (MAS). The most common way of assessing this is to cover a distance of 1.6km as fast as possible. Then divide the distance in metres by the time it takes to complete the distance in seconds. For example, player A completed the 1.6km in 6 minutes (320 seconds). The calculation of 1600/320 gives a total of 4.4. Therefore, the MAS is 4.4ms. If you want to train at this aerobic speed, you must not exceed the value of 4.4 metres per second. This training method was originated by Tabata et al. (1996), and subsequently modified within team sports by Baker (2011), who proposes 15 seconds on, 15 seconds off at the MAS for greater aerobic adaptations. Calculating/quantifying intensity of maximal speed work can be done with less complicated scientific methods.

Furthermore, those coaches working with sprint athletes, or those coaches delivering specific speed work with their athletes can use percentage of maximal speed, attained by a timed sprint, or from GPS data and so on. The percentage would then potentially change between repetitions of warm up sets and maximal speed work so an average percentage can then be calculated as the session intensity figure. As mentioned with intensity quantification, techniques such as RPE or a coach's scale can be implemented with physiological/maximal speed intensity, so coaches working with little technology can

31

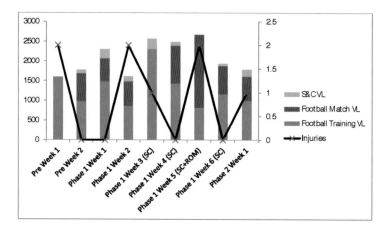

Weekly volume loads (total minutes × RPE) within an elite athlete squad. Volume loads are broken down within the week to gym-based, field, and competitive matches. This provides a tool that is cheap and time efficient if no others are available. However, other precise measures should be used in conjunction within the gym and field training. Numbers of injuries are plotted against the graph to see if there is a link between the volume load completed and breakdown. Quite often, it is the weeks before the injury that occurred that are likely to cause the injury (if overload). However, there were only two 'overload' injuries within the seven recorded here. Note that the number of injuries doesn't tell you the nature or severity of the injuries; it is therefore imperative that greater injury description is provided and looked into.

Rating of Percieved Exertion (RPE Scale)	
10	Maximal
9	Really, Really Hard
8	Really Hard
7	
6	Hard
5	Challenging
4	Moderate
3	Easy
2	Really Easy
1	Rest

The RPE chart shown to athletes post-session to obtain their RPE score, which would be calculated with duration.

provide an efficient quantification of intensity also (Turner *et al.*, 2014).

PUTTING VOLUME AND INTENSITY INTO A PROGRAMME

Previously discussed were the various ways in which volume and intensity may be calculated within our working environment; now a programme with calculated volume and intensity can be constructed. From both a training adaptation and injury prevention perspective, it is the fluctuation of volume and intensity that is essential (Stone *et al.*, 1999a; 1999b). There is no clear way of fluctuating volume and intensity, although strong recommendations can be made on the structure of it. For example, looking at a team sport where competition is weekly, the volume might be increased to the middle of the week at its maximum, and then reduced prior to the game, to optimize the freshness of the athlete

(Chadd, 2010). The same rule can be applied for longer macro cycles and sports with more sporadic competitions. However, within the monthly schedule of any sport, there must be fluctuation also in what is prescribed weekly. Furthermore, there might be within a four-week cycle a linear increase in volume of work, with a significant reduction in week four as an overall recovering week (Plisk and Stone, 2003). This is a basic concept that obviously has to fit the needs and requirements of each sport and yearly calendar, but it must be stressed that an athlete cannot follow the same loading week after week in a team sport in an attempt to maximize their freshness for every game. (An athlete will never be 100 per cent fresh for every game – even though they will never know this.) Attempting to do this will see greater reductions in performance over the season and greater risk of injury (Siff, 2003). Several weeks therefore should be targeted as essential weeks of 100 per cent freshness; others will be weeks where the load is higher to drive adaptation in a desired physical quality or qualities. This will reduce injury risk over time and attempt to enhance our athletes' various physical qualities over a year, where the off-season and pre-season is so short. In sports where competition is more sporadic or occurs in a short time period (athletics or swimming for example), it is potentially easier to plan an athlete to peak at certain times, although some competitions will be targeted when an athlete will not be 100 per cent and the expectation is therefore lower. This is essential and necessary for maximal freshness at selected competitions.

Two examples of a particular high force phase are given in visual form in the two graphs. The athlete completing these programmes was a football player, and this was the resistance programme, running in conjunction to his technical/tactical training. The first graph demonstrates the total volume and intensity of work in each week within the monthly cycle. As evident, there is a three-

week gradual increase in both volume and intensity, remembering that overload is essential for greater adaptation (Baechle and Earle, 2000). Week three would therefore be deemed as the the week with most adaptation, when the athlete would be placed under greatest physiological (or mechanical) load. Week four, however, demonstrates a reduction in both volume and intensity to allow a de-load or recovery week, to ensure the

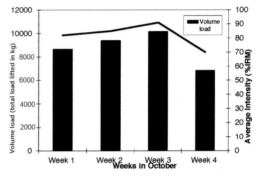

An example resistance weekly loading session within a monthly cycle. Volume and intensity are demonstrated. Weekly loads are the combination of two resistance sessions within this athlete's weekly schedule.

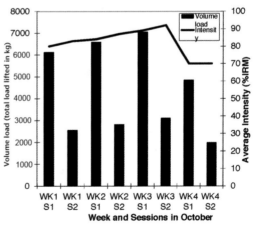

The same monthly cycle, with a visual breakdown of volume and intensity within each resistance session.

adaptation occurs and the athlete is kept as fresh as possible. (It is also essential to note that at the end of week four was a very important game against potential contenders for the title, so the importance of peaking for that particular game was a priority.) As a general rule, although load should be managed throughout the week, tailored towards weekly matches, it must be stressed that trying to ensure your athletes maintain the same freshness levels each week is virtually impossible, and load on a weekly basis needs to be altered. This is clearly evident in the second graph where you can see a breakdown of volume and intensity for each session throughout the monthly cycle. As you can see, within each week volume in particular is reduced for the session closest to the game so a level of freshness is restored and fatigue is reduced. However, the same pattern occurs with an increase in volume for three weeks combined with a general de-load week. It is important to understand this, as it clearly demonstrates a new approach in periodization for sports such as football: the same weekly load is not prescribed week after week.

It is important to note that there is a significant trade-off with high volumes of training load, however it is quantified. High training volumes – not intensity – have been demonstrated to be significantly correlated with higher injury rates. The optimal load for each individual athlete is unknown, and becomes guesswork in the applied setting, even for the best strength and conditioning coaches. However, higher volumes are essential for greater gains in performance; it is therefore essential to change the focus of a particular phase, so that a particular training volume is directed into different physical priorities, fluctuating the load further within the cycle as evident in the graphs above. Although it seems that lower training volumes would seem optimal for reducing injury rates, the athlete will become de-conditioned and could increase their injury risk within

competition, as well as not reaching their physical genetic ceiling. They need to be able to sustain a variety of different training volumes, but the S&C coach should be clever in the phasic approach to optimize adaptations and minimize injury.

A fascinating article by Blagrove (2014) in the March issue of the UKSCA Journal highlights a very good approach to periodizing physical programmes within team sports where the off-season is short, and physical qualities need to be enhanced throughout the competitive season. (It must be noted that sports that have few competitive dates within the calendar year, or those that cycle towards an Olympic event can arguably use an effective linear periodization, which can be easier to plan.) In my experience working within team organizations, I have seen a number of periodized plans; although they have all offered completely contrasting philosophies, they have in my opinion been very similar in the overall periodization strategy. Here an undulated periodization approach was taken, where many physical, technical and tactical qualities were prescribed over the training week. Although the foundations of this work seem logical, there are flaws if the programme offers little variety and no change of emphasis over the season. Blagrove's article suggests that certain physical qualities need to be highlighted and emphasized at certain times whilst others are reduced. This way certain physical qualities are saturated whilst others are maintained. This provides a well thought out approach to considering the overall load the athlete is going through, a greater variety and a lack of monotony, which can be another precursor for overload injuries.

DAILY MONITORING TOOLS WITHIN AN ELITE ENVIRONMENT

Within my personal experience, working with

some fantastic sports scientists, monitoring tools have been an essential aspect of their role to prepare athletes for daily training, reducing injury potential and keeping them performing to the highest standard possible. Subsequently, I have identified two very effective methods of monitoring fatigue levels in athletes. The first method consists of an objective measure of fatigue, more precisely neuromuscular fatigue in measuring the reactive strength index (RSI) from a drop jump exercise. Although neuromuscular fatigue isn't measured directly, the jump test is suggested to be a good indicator. RSI can be calculated by jump height/contact time (Flanagan and Comyns, 2008), although flight time can also be used. It has been discovered firstly that RSI is significantly decreased after soccer sporting activity, therefore can represent a reliable and valid level of the neuromuscular fatigue within sporting activity (Oliver, Armstrong, and Williams, 2008).

RSI has been traditionally measured by a force platform, which is extremely expensive and impractical for the majority of sporting clubs/organizations, although it would increase the validity of results. A portable contact jump mat may be used; this has proven to be very reliable and valid for the use of calculating RSI (Lloyd et al. 2009). Athletes would perform a drop jump test, or three tests, and either the best one or average is taken, measuring RSI first thing in the morning when they report to duties. Their score will then be compared to a baseline RSI score attained when the athletes are fresh; it must be noted that the baseline scores should be updated every 4–6 weeks to account for training adaptation. A comparison of their daily jump can then be made, determining their current fatigue level. Hopkins (2004), a well-known guru within sports statistics, suggested that within power measures, a decrease in RSI of 0.2 standard deviations (SD) below baseline would represent a trivial difference, a decrease between 0.2 and 0.6 SD would be a small difference, 0.6–1.2 SD a moderate difference, and 1.2–2.0 SD below representing a large difference. This type of data then allows the coach to assess the severity of fatigue the player is currently experiencing from previous bouts of training

Short questionnaire on fatigue

The previous session/since the previous session:						
1	I have found training more difficult than usual	1	2	3	4	5
2	I have not eaten or drunk very well	1	2	3	4	5
3	I have not slept very well	1	2	3	4	5
4	My legs felt/feel sore/heavy	1	2	3	4	5
5	I have a sore throat/runny nose/cold/infection/flu	1	2	3	4	5
6	I felt/feel more anxious/irritable than usual	1	2	3	4	5
7	I had/have more stress at home/school/training than usual	1	2	3	4	5
8	I felt/feel less motivated to train today than usual	1	2	3	4	5
Sum of short questionnaire on fatigue						
1= Totally Disagree; 2= Somewhat Disagree; 3= Normal; 4= Somewhat Agree; 5= Totally Agree						

or competition. It then allows the coach – depending on the level of fatigue, or how many days the athlete has been below their baseline level – to make a decision on potentially modifying their training loads. If athletes are below their threshold for more than three days in a row, they are significantly more likely to break down or become injured, although this is a practical observation, not a scientific finding. As ever, it is a balancing act: at times, being suppressed and fatigued is inevitable due to training overload/overreaching phases, which are essential for adaptation. Once again, knowing how much load an athlete can tolerate before sufficient recovery is essential is key to the modification required.

There is another, more subjective, tool of monitoring which can be equally effective and supplement the objective data from the RSI scores. A questionnaire to the athletes in the morning also provides essential information about fatigue. Questions include topics around the last training session, sleep, soreness, motivation, nutrition, etc. This method provides an effective, holistic approach to understanding the state of the athlete and how fatigue and overtraining can be avoided (Turner *et al.*, 2014).

RECOVERY STRATEGIES

The second part of this chapter will assess a topic that is a focus at almost every applied sporting organization and club in the world: utilizing effective recovery strategies. Applying an external stimulus to the body is often done post-competition or training session to enhance the recovery of the athlete, leading to greater training and performance quality, as well as a reduction in injury. There are many techniques available to the practitioner, with varying financial cost. These techniques will be discussed in turn, with a brief review of the literature, also taking into account personal experiences within the field and discussing how effective various recovery strategies really are. Recovery strategies are most commonly used within team sports that have weekly competitive fixtures; sports that compete less frequently generally have time to recover naturally post competition, and would only use recovery strategies for recovery during competition or potentially a high load training phase.

Warm-downs

Many sports clubs and athletes will perform some form of 'warm-down' post competition or training. Stretching will not be discussed in this section, as increasing range of movement will be discussed in Chapter 3); this section will focus on performing active recovery post-exercise. It has been documented that active recovery is greater than passive recovery, with greater reduction in lactate levels and a higher resynthesis of glycogen in a 60-minute period (Choi *et al.*, 1994), mainly attributable to a quicker clearance of lactate from the muscles and blood. (Remember that although lactate isn't responsible for fatigue, it does provide a good indicator that high amounts of acidity and hydrogen ions are present, which would suggest greater fatigue.) It must also be noted however, that lactate levels return to normal resting values after approximately 90 minutes in amphibians (Gleeson, 1982) and 2 hours in humans (Gaesser and Brooks, 1984), without any intervention post-exercise. This research has been conclusive for some time now – these studies were conducted over thirty years ago – so the misconception that active recovery can enhance lactate removal within a day is baffling. Therefore, unless a second training session or competition is being performed within a 2-hour period, the active recovery approach will have little effect on lactate removal and restoration of pH levels.

Reilly and Rigby (2002) conducted a study that reported findings in one group that completed a warm-down post-exercise, and another group that didn't. They measured various performance parameters post-exercise and over a 72-hour period. It was discovered that there was a lower reduction in performance in the recovery group, and resting parameters were restored quicker, providing the need for warm-downs within an athlete's schedule. However, there was no mechanistic or physiological difference in any markers assessed, which provides a potential argument that a psychological effect took place. This trend seems to occur in the majority of the studies regarding warm-downs, and that there is no physiological mechanism that can explain an enhanced recovery. From experience, athletes feel better in themselves and less 'tight' or 'stiff' when performing a warm-down post-competition in particular, even if the quality of the warm-down is poor. Therefore, eliciting a psychological effect for athletes when prescribing a warm-down could provide a sufficient rationale, even though there is little science to support it.

Sports massage

Massage techniques are used in many sports as a therapeutic and sometimes more aggressive way of enhancing athletes' recovery. The benefits that are proposed for the use of massage with athletes include improving stretching of tendons and connective structures and therefore relieving muscle tension by relieving a trigger point within the muscle (Ryan, 1980: Stamford, 1985), as well as a possible increase in blood flow which in turn enhances lactate removal (Ylinen and Cash, 1988). The effect of enhancing lactate removal was previously discussed, providing doubt over that theory of enhancing recovery. Although these theories have been proposed and many practitioners still believe in them, there has been very little scientific evidence to support them. For example, a more recent study from Hemmings

et al. (2010) assessed the possible effect massage had on the recovery of repeated boxing exercise. Many physiological markers were assessed but no difference was found between the two different groups. However, there was a significant difference between perceived recovery of those who had massage intervention and those who didn't, therefore providing further evidence that a psychological benefit is gained from this recovery technique for the athlete.

One new alternative massage type involves the new foam roller: a piece of portable equipment that athletes can manipulate by themselves, to create a massage effect in particular muscle groups. There is, however, very little research (if any) on the effective use of this piece of equipment. In my opinion this would have a very similar outcome as the massage itself; even though it has a more superficial effect on the muscles, it is based on the same principle of myofascial release and trigger points. Furthermore, although its physiological effects are questioned within applied practice it does provide a potential psychological stimulus to the athletes, and increases their perceived range of movement at particular muscles and joints. It also provides a logistical and financial benefit in comparison to traditional massage by a professional.

Cold water immersion

Cold water immersion (CWI), commonly known as an 'ice bath', has been used for recovery for many years. The scientific theory behind it is that it causes a reduction in tissue temperature post-exercise, which can affect blood flow and cause a decrease in the inflammatory response caused by oxidative stress of the exercise bout (White and Wells, 2013). An interesting review was published by Bleakley and Davison (2010), which analysed particular studies that met certain criteria: only studies that used temperatures below 15 degrees Celsius and five-minute durations were included. This was proposed as there is conclusive evidence that cold water immersion bouts of longer duration – up to ten minutes – can have a physiological effect on recovery. Therefore, it was essential to assess the effect of shorter bouts of cold water immersion. However, the common trend from this study proposed a similar outcome to those of other recovery strategy research: although there was a perceived recovery increase from the athlete, there was no physiological change from the shorter bout of CWI. It is concluded that around 10 degrees Celsius has been proposed the optimal water temperature for cold water immersion.

It has also been suggested that the physiological response due to a CWI stimulus is not because of the temperature, but the pressure of the water (White and Wells, 2013). Therefore, greater benefits would be elicited in a bath of height, where the whole body is covered and the pressure is the greatest. This however, needs further research to be conclusive. Although there is some scientific evidence that there is a physiological response from CWI, it is important to understand that it can blunt the inflammatory response caused by the training stress (White and Wells, 2013). This inflammatory response, however, is an important process of adaptation (Blennerhassett et al., 1992), and by stopping this natural response to exercise, it could elicit a reduction in physiological adaptation. Further views on this will be outlined later; however, it must be said that caution should be taken if using CWI recovery techniques on a regular training basis as desired training adaptation could be hindered.

Reviewing the recovery strategies presented above, it is clear that a common theme is presented when scientifically researching these modalities. For example, the only recovery strategy that provides a physiological change identified in research is cold water immersion that immerses the whole body for a duration of longer than 5 minutes. The rest of the recovery techniques seem to elicit only a feeling of perceived recovery from the athletes without any physiological change. From experience, if it gives the athlete a feeling of perceived freshness, then there is no problem with the strategies being put in place. However, the expense of such strategies should be taken into account; an inexpensive foam roller which athletes can use themselves when they wish, without the expense of a therapist's cost or time, might be preferable. The CWI strategy, if structured well, can have a benefit on recovery, although the potential issue noted above (the reduction of the inflammatory response having a potentially negative impact on adaptation) should be remembered; this strategy is therefore recommended within a competition phase, where a number of games are played in a short time frame, such as a world cup in various sports, or Olympic Games, but its use should be limited within a training period. As discussed previously, the periodization should be structured well, and allow for sufficient recovery from training, without the use of recovery strategies. The inflammatory response and training fatigue is a necessary requirement for enhancement and adaptation of a physical quality. What is an effective strategy in terms of recovery and essential for performance is nutritional intake, including fluids, and this will be discussed in the next section.

Restoration of energy

When an athlete completes a 'hard' training session physiologically, some glycogen depletion will have taken place (Ekblom, 1986: 2002), and therefore there may be physical and cognitive impairments (Reilly and Ekblom, 2005). It is essential that a restoration of energy is completed for recovery of the athlete prior to the next session or competition. The optimal time of replenishment is said to be within the first two hours of cessation of exercise as glycogen synthesis is highest (Ivy *et al.*, 1988). There is also evidence of potential increased glucose sensitivity and GLUT 4 immediately post-exercise (Dohm, 2002). Nutritional guidelines suggest a carbohydrate intake of 1.5g/kg of body weight post-exercise, which would be 120g of carbohydrates for an 80kg athlete. However, this has been proposed to have limitations as it has been suggested that anything over 50g of carbohydrates proposes no extra benefit than added unnecessary calories (Coyle, 1991), which in turn could be detrimental to body composition. Although appetite can often be suppressed post-exercise, a liquid form beverage high in glycogen would be sufficient initially before a meal later on.

It is also well known that for optimal recovery, a carbohydrate mixed with protein and amino acids enhances all-round recovery, due to an increase in protein synthesis post-exercise (Ramussen *et al.*, 2000). It is stressed that a net protein gain is essential, otherwise there could be degradation of energy stores and musculature function, due to athletes being in a catabolic state (Tipton and Wolfe, 2001). It is interesting to note, however, like the carbohydrate limit, there is no benefit from exceeding over approximately 20–30g of protein post-exercise (precisely 0.25g/kg of bodyweight), and anything over that amount would be excreted and therefore wasted. The process of replenishing stress should also be continued the next day and an extra 8–10g/kg should be taken over the day, ensuring 60 per cent of the diet is carbohydrates. However, it must be stressed that this method and volume of carbohydrate should be adopted only if a high intensity/volume session or training phase has been completed, and even pre-competition. In my experience sports such as football, rugby, and hockey rarely need this extreme high amount of carbohydrates, and consumption would cause negative effects. It is therefore up to the practitioner to assess the requirements of their athletes based on the demands and how hard the training phase is.

There is a recent trend, a combination of the Paleo diet and the work of Professor Tim Noakes: the low carbohydrate, high fat (LCHF) diet, which, it is suggested, is far more beneficial to athletes than the traditional high-carbohydrate athlete diet. It is proposed that due to the high GI of many grains and high-carbohydrate-based food there will be a high glycogen spike and consequently an insulin response, which is detrimental to function and athletic performance. Also, a higher fat and protein diet would enable the athlete to switch their main fuel utilization to fats and protein, which would be more efficient and significantly advantageous for body composition. However, in my experience, for athletic performance carbohydrates should not be eliminated altogether. They should be cycled and fluctuated depending on the phase but should still remain a main aspect of an athlete's dietary intake.

Rehydration

During strenuous competition core body temperature has been demonstrated to rise above 39 degrees Celsius (Ekblom, 1986), although core temperature is influenced by both exercise intensity and environmental factors. When core temperature rises, the body naturally sweats to cool the body down, leading to a loss of fluids from the body. The loss of fluids has been demonstrated to impair technical and physical performance if not replaced (Burke and Ekblom, 1982). It must be remembered that water alone cannot replace the lost salts from the body; therefore an electrolyte drink is suggested post-competition, and even during competition at certain intervals, if accessible. Interestingly, if electrolyte losses are not restored, much of the water absorption is lost again through urination, emphasizing the need for an electrolyte-based solution post-competition.

From experience, coaches need to be aware of athletes over-using electrolyte drinks in a normal day, as they are heavily marketed as a product that is 'good for you'. Stress to athletes that these should be used only for rehydration and restoring of minerals post-competition or after training; excessive use of them could lead to unnecessary weight gain due to their high calorie content.

Hydration should be monitored regularly for the education of the athlete, and optimal scores should be highlighted. Optimal hydration scores should be reported as 200–600, which correlates to lighter-coloured urine. It is proposed that being in a euhydrated state can actually impair repeated sprint ability and force production (Van Winckel *et al*., 2014), which highlights the lower hydration score, below 100 (measured by the osmolality of the urine) isn't always optimal for performance.

The section above has given a concise overview of the nutritional aspects of recovery; a strength and conditioning coach may not necessarily have the time to delve into nutritional protocols in too much detail, but the reader is directed to a review by Maughan and Shirreffs (2000), which displays a good overview of nutritional intake post-exercise for nutrition, although there are many other detailed reviews on this topic area within the current literature.

As discussed within this chapter, there are many techniques and strategies available to enhance the recovery of an athlete in-between training bouts and/or prior to competition. A pattern emerged with many of the strategies that there is little scientific evidence to back them up physiologically, and most rely on a having a positive psychological impact on the athlete. Consequently, it is my view that a high budget and reliance on recovery strategies is unnecessary. Instead, the practitioner should focus on well-structured periodization, optimal nutrition and good quality and quantity of sleep. If these variables are performed correctly with other training parameters then the athlete will be in a strong position to stay injury-free.

3 | RANGE OF MOVEMENT AND CORRECTIVE EXERCISE

The range of movement (ROM) an athlete has depends on each particular joint, and a variety of genetic/anthropometric and training history factors. This chapter will look to enhance the knowledge of the practitioner, in increasing the range of movement of an athlete and its effect on injury prevention. ROM is often termed 'mobility' or 'flexibility', although within the context of this book, mobility will be used to describe the range of movement at particular joints in a dynamic movement, whereas flexibility will be used to describe the ROM in a static way. These two methods and the differences will be explained in further detail but it must be known that these terms are often used interchangeably in the relevant literature.

Increasing ROM or having a large ROM has been proposed for many years in the sporting environment as a predetermining factor to a reduction in injury potential (Kibler *et al.*, 1996; Myers *et al.*, 2006). Increasing ROM and performing certain modalities post-exercise have been proposed to reduce delayed onset muscle soreness, commonly known as DOMS – (Cleak and Eston, 1992), although very little scientific evidence has proved that. There is more conclusive evidence that a lack of ROM may not have such a big impact on an acute injury to that area, but will contribute to more overload injuries due to high compensation at another joint (Clark and Lucett, 2010). What has become apparent over the last few years is that performing different types of activities to enhance range of movement should be done at different times, and taking a more dynamic approach in general is what athletes need to start doing to alter mobility characteristics and prevent injury (Starrett, 2013).

In my experience, there are three main areas of mobility concern within athletes: the ankle, hip, and thoracic spine. A lack of mobility at these joints can cause issues at other joints due to other areas over-compensating to achieve a movement. For many athletes, ensuring they are mobile in all of these joints will create a better mover. Here is a rough model that the athletes I am currently working with follow:

1. Self myofascial release (with a foam roller) of any tight muscles, regulating any neurological pathways.
2. Stretching any tight muscles (stretching should be limited on days when high force/velocity work is being performed in the gym).
3. Mobilizing the required joints in both a static and dynamic manipulation before

an integrated squatting and lunging pattern.

It is then the duty of the coach to ensure the range is tested through a variety of various functional movements, testing the range at

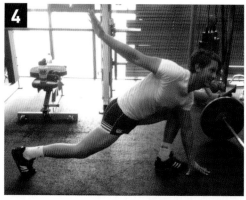

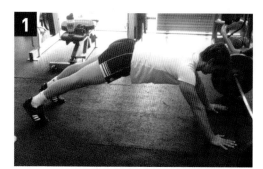

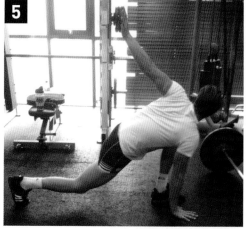

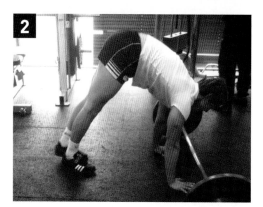

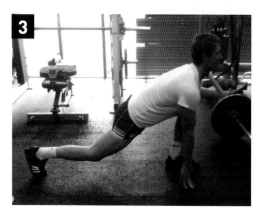

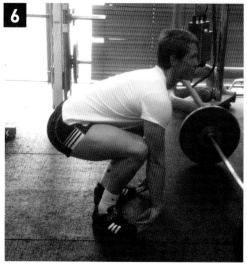

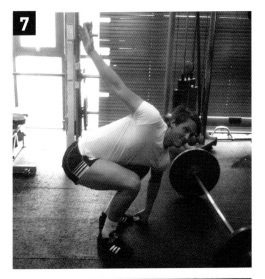

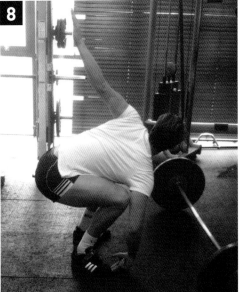

each joint through various directions and so on. It is important that these measures are tested through FMS tests, but also through manual manipulation tests at the various joints to provide an objective measure of ROM. Measure ankle and hip movement with a goniometer; effective communication and collaboration with the physiotherapist is essential in assessing results.

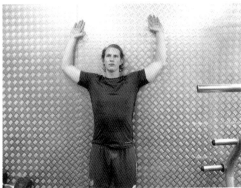

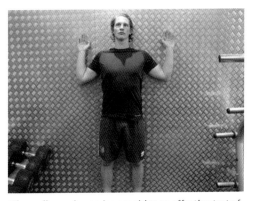

These exercises enhance the mobility of athletes in a dynamic/functional movement. The first exercise (1 and 2), termed the 'inchworm', enhances hamstring flexibility and mobility at the hips. The lunge (3, 4 and 5) and squat (6, 7 and 8) exercises aim to enhance both ankle and hip mobility, cuing as much as depth as possible. However, the two exercises also include a thoracic rotation to enhance thoracic mobility.

The wall angel exercise provides an effective test of thoracic mobility and scapula activation. Ensure every part of the body is touching a wall, make an angel movement and see how much ROM the thoracic spine allows.

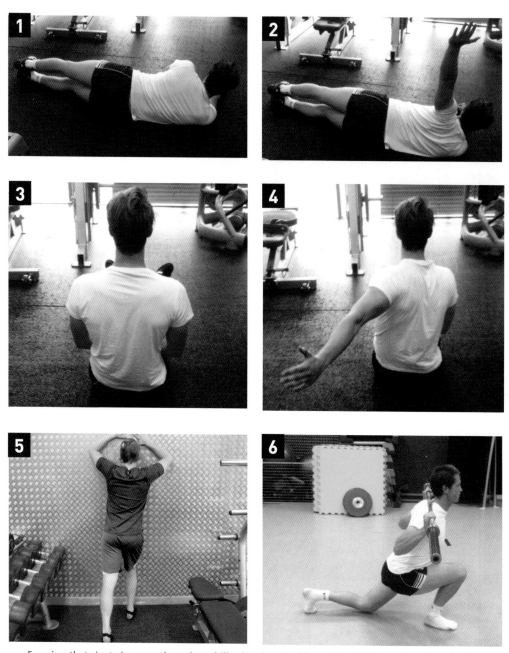

Exercises that aim to increase thoracic mobility (1–4) and ankle mobility (5), increasing dorsiflexion. Encourage the athlete with the knee to wall to move the foot back as they progress, and to go through static and dynamic movements. The split squat/lunge exercises (6) encourage greater dorsiflexion in a dynamic exercise.

WARM-UPS AND THE INFLUENCE OF ROM

For many years there has been much controversy over the optimal warm-up within the research and applied field. It was traditionally held that athletes must static stretch prior to competition or any exercise modality to prevent injury to a muscle. However, in more recent years this has become viewed as a modality that not only lacks scientific evidence for injury prevention, but could also potentially have a negative effect on performance. Much research demonstrates that static stretching can acutely decrease power output and high force/velocity performance (Marek, Cramer and Culkertson, 2005), although Power *et al.* (2004) found a decrease in force and torque production, but contrastingly, no decrease in jump performance. There is evidence supporting both arguments, and nothing is set in stone in terms of performance, although clear evidence that static stretching pre-exercise reduces the risk of injury is lacking.

Further review of the literature and greater detail regarding static stretching are given later on in this chapter. Static stretching would of course increase the flexibility of muscles or joints as a general modality, and this will be discussed later in the chapter also. Prior to exercise, warm-ups should incorporate a phase of mobilization, which includes increasing the ROM of particular joints and muscles in a dynamic way, preferably in similar patterns to those that would occur in that sport. Exercises could include dynamic leg swings and their variations for the hip and knee joints, some walking/running mechanic drills that can include the dorsi- and plantarflexion of the ankle, and range of movement at the shoulder joint if required. It is proposed that these dynamic exercises are preferred before exercise as they replicate the movements that would be required in performance more than static stretches. It is essential that within these exercises athletes are strongly encouraged to take the movement to the full ROM for optimal benefit. If available, there are many hurdle drills that can be done for an increasing ROM purpose, prior to training/competition if logistically possible or within an individual session with the aim of increasing mobility.

It is interesting to note that mobilization exercises can also be combined with activation exercises within a warm-up; exercises such as bodyweight squats and lunges are good examples of this. Although not directly within the chapter of ROM, this seems a good point at which to propose a basic warm-up structure coaches can apply and adapt to their athlete and sport. The proposed warm-up protocol will follow the 'RAMP' method, first proposed by Jeffreys (2007), editor of the UKSCA Journal and board member. The warm-up is also a prime opportunity to coach players within certain movements, as an S&C coach's time with an athlete is often limited.

Raiser

Increase heart rate, core temperature, breathing rate, etc. Physiological activation of energy systems.

Activation

Look to activate key musculature prior to performance. For example, the most common muscles activated prior to training/competition are the posterior chain and the glutes (as discussed in previous chapters), and the shoulder stabilizing muscles. This does depend on the sporting requirements, however.

Mobilization

As previously discussed, increasing ROM of

Phase of warm-up	Content	Time
Raiser	Various locomotor patterns (jog/skip/shuffle, etc.) Low intensity technical work with football	8 mins
Activation	Glute bridges Band work (isolation) BW squats BW lunges (integration)	8 mins
	Dynamic leg swings Hip mobility drills	
Mobilization		
Technical and physiological intensity increase	Possession game with overload for attacking team	2 × 5 mins
Specific position technical work	Player-specific technical work according to position	5 mins
Potentiation	Reaction to stimulus – maximal sprinting and jumping	3 mins
		Total time of warm-up including breaks, transition, etc.: 35–40 minutes

joints and muscles. Can be prescribed with exercises that only increase ROM or can be combined with activation exercises.

Potentiation

Increasing the neurological function, and performing some exercises that significantly increase the intensity up to maximal. Examples of maximal sprints and jumps are most common modalities used in this section.

Low-level technical work can be incorporated into the raiser section, whereas higher intensity work should be performed after the activation/mobilization phases, prior to the potentiation, which should always be the very last stage performed. Even in endurance events maximal work that activates neural systems can enhance performance. An example from a warm-up completed on a match day of an elite football club prior to competition is demonstrated in the table.

The warm-up above should provide a template that is accessible for coaches, and can be adapted and modified to each particular sport. It must be noted that this is not the only warm-up template available and practitioners are urged to find one that works for their players and optimizes their performance.

Although slightly outside the topic area of this chapter, it is important to discuss the intensity level of the warm-up. There are two opposing concepts within the research/ applied sporting world with regard to the intensity of warm ups. Firstly, research from the infamous Aspire Academy in Qatar has demonstrated that if intensity goes above 80 per cent VO2 max, a reduction in glycogen occurs, which could negatively impact sporting performance. However, it is also demonstrated that a warm-up requires an athlete to go over their lactate threshold, which can occur anywhere between 50–80 per cent of VO2 max, due to athlete variability. This is due to an enhanced VO2 kinetics, acutely increasing physiological performance. Therefore, to combat glycogen depletion, and still maintain a high-intensity warm up, glycogen supplements should be administered in the forms of gels, drinks etc.

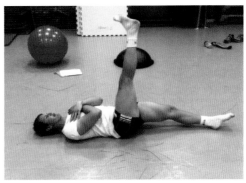

An example of an active stretch of the hamstrings. Evidently this type of stretch has limitations, as the range of stretch possible is limited.

As you can see in the warm-up template above, there is no time allotted for static stretching. Not only is this due to the lack of scientific evidence around the benefits of static stretching, but also due to evidence that static stretching can negatively impact explosive performance. Power *et al.* (2004) demonstrated that even a moderate stretching routine caused a decrease in torque production from the quadriceps on an isokinetic dynamometer. Behm and Chaouachi (2011) provide a fascinating review on the topic area and offer a collection of studies that demonstrate reductions in strength, jump, and speed performances with stretching protocols as little as two minutes, although it is suggested that longer stretching times cause a greater decrease in performance. The aim of this textbook is not to delve into the mechanical details of why this occurs but it has been demonstrated that static stretching causes a negative neurological deficit in the speed of signals sent, reducing the force and velocity of contraction. Although there are studies that do not show a decrease in performance, there is enough evidence to suggest that it could have a damaging effect on high force/velocity tasks, and it is therefore not recommended within a warm-up.

The biggest challenge within elite sport, however, is to change the thought processes of particular athletes. If static stretching has always been done within their warm-up routine, then they are often very reluctant to take it out. Therefore, give them a period of time within the warm-up to perform static stretching if they require it, but don't make it a regimented part of the warm-up. This way, its importance will start to reduce in the athlete's eyes. Further, if the time spent static stretching can be reduced or kept as short as possible, this could decrease the negative effect it can have on performance. If less and less time is allotted on static stretching over time, it may be possible to phase it out completely. A similar thing was done by me, with both static stretching and warm-downs, as neither modalities have a proven advantageous effect on injury prevention or recovery. However, static stretching post-exercise can be beneficial and is something that is used in my practice. It's not used as a warm-down/recovery tool but for increasing ROM at certain joints. Stretching modalities will be discussed later, although it should be emphasized here that long durations and stretching past normal ROM are essential for adaptation. In my opinion, stretching programmes are not performed aggressively enough and consequently adaptation is very limited. The sport of gymnastics, although it came under substantial criticism for its methods, particularly within Chinese traditions, provides a good indication of the pain and aggressiveness of stretching required for maximizing adaptation to increase ROM and flexibility. The three types of static stretching that will be discussed are active, passive, and proprioceptive neuromuscular facilitation (PNF).

Active stretching

This type of stretching is when only the agonist muscle being stretched provides the movement with no other external influences. For example, when an athlete lays on their back and brings their leg straight up in the air to stretch the hamstrings, there is no use of anything other than the leg muscles to hold the stretch. This example of an active stretch is questionable in terms of aggressiveness and effectiveness and, in my opinion, has limited use when attempting to increase ROM.

Passive stretching

This stretching allows an external stimulus to apply a greater stretch – the environment, equipment, or another person. For example, if the same stretch is performed in the active stretch then a partner could apply more pressure to the stretch to take it past the natural ROM, enhancing adaptation. This modality would be an essential starting point for static stretching and has potential for the greatest adaptation in ROM and flexibility. Another technique that can be applied within the passive stretching technique is to use the environment for a greater ROM. For example, the hamstrings stretch where an athlete is sitting on the ground and tries to reach further with their hands utilizes the ground to keep a fully extended lower limb. This type of stretch, commonly seen in Chinese gymnastics, not

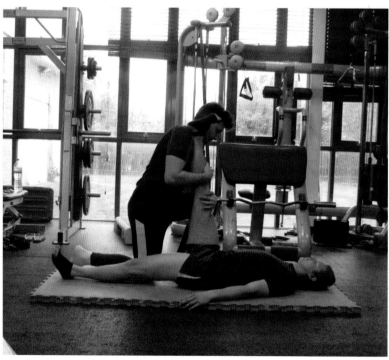

The same hamstrings stretch being performed in a passive/PNF way. With passive pressure greater range is achieved and neural adaptations can occur (as discussed in PNF stretching). With all stretching modalities, ensure that the lower back is in neutral position and the stretch comes from 'loose' hips.

only utilizes the ground but also an external force in a coach, forcing the athlete even further. This is an aggressive example of static stretching – one that would see greater adaptation, although it creates more discomfort. This type of stretching has come under heavy criticism and this book by no means endorses this type of aggression and discomfort with this age group. However, it does provide a clear example of the aggression that can be placed within stretching routines.

Proprioceptive neuromuscular facilitation (PNF)

This type of stretching has been proposed to be most effective in ROM gains. It consists of a phase of passive stretching, coupled with some isometric contractions of that muscle area, a period of relaxation and then a further increase of ROM in a second bout of passive stretching. It is most commonly used in the hamstrings stretch demonstrated in the passive stretching example, where the athlete is on their back being stretched by a partner. It is important that the isometric contraction is done maximally, to increase the neural drive and override the stretch reflex from the muscle spindles and Golgi tendon organs (GTO), which act as a protective mechanism. There are many time protocols that are proposed for this technique, although a standard time frame would be a passive stretch for 20 seconds, 10 seconds of isometric contraction, 10 seconds of recovery and a further 20 seconds of passive stretching. However, progression is important and as well as increasing ROM, increasing the time under tension is another important method for optimizing adaptation.

There are other names and types of stretch in addition to those described above, though these are the most commonly used modalities. Active stretching is not the preferred option in my opinion, due to lack of aggression and ability to push the stretch further than its

typical ROM. Passive and PNF in particular are better examples of a more aggressive approach to static stretching and increasing ROM.

Ensure that when static stretching is performed there is no over-compensation with any other area. For example, when sitting down or standing to stretch the hamstrings by trying to touch their toes, often athletes use the curving of their lower back (lumbar region) to stretch further. This not only defeats the object of trying to maximize the stretch of the hamstrings and increase hip mobility, but causes curvature of the lumbar spine, a position not desirable for the fully functional athlete. This point will be further discussed in the next section on testing ROM and incorporating that into sessions.

....

CORRECTIVE EXERCISE

Testing ROM: influencing good practice

A common flexibility test performed in schools, sporting clubs and organizations is what is known as the 'sit and reach' test, which specifically tests the flexibility of the hamstrings. As mentioned briefly, the problem with this is that athletes can achieve a greater score in terms of distance of stretch due to a further curvature of the spine and not greater flexibility in the hamstrings. This again, provides inaccurate results in the flexibility of the hamstrings, but also sends the misleading message to athletes that curvature of the spine is acceptable; even if it is unloaded and not dangerous, it is poor practice in the training of the trunk and hip mobility. Instead, a flexibility test of the hamstrings should consist of a hip hinge type of exercise. This would require the hamstrings to be fixed and fully extended, whilst the movement of the hip ensures good posture is kept at the lumbar region and the full range of that athlete is achieved. Obviously, this technical model requires some training and familiarization of the exercise before testing; however, it provides a much more realistic functional test of hip mobility and flexibility of the hamstrings.

Other tests that are much more functional look at the mobility of a joint in more of a dynamic way. A good indicator to highlight this would to assess an athlete's standing hip flexion before the lumbar spine cannot hold a neutral position any more. This can be hard to implement, however, and there are easier assessments available. For example, the Functional Movement Screen (Cook, 2010) and variations are very good assessments of how an athlete can move, even though the scores are very subjective. Modifications of the FMS in my opinion are very useful, and if you as a practitioner can come up with particular exercises and movements that you think are useful and relevant then it can be a great assessment tool. The overhead squat is another great exercise to prescribe: it provides visual information on the athlete's shoulder mobility/stability, mobility and stability at the three lower limb joints, and the ability of the trunk to stabilize the movement. With this exercise, the guideline states that an athlete's stance must be shoulder-width apart. Although within training you might advise adopting a wider stance, the narrow stance during this testing allows any compensation to be magnified and highlighted.

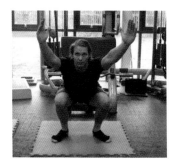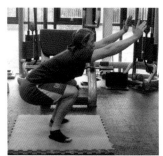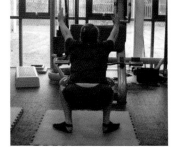

Subject A: Overhead squat screen.

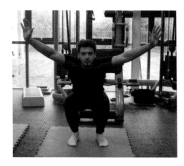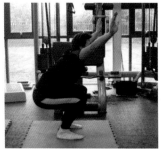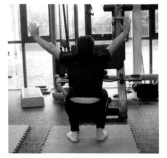

Subject B: Overhead squat screen.

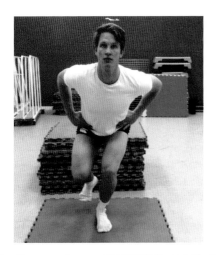

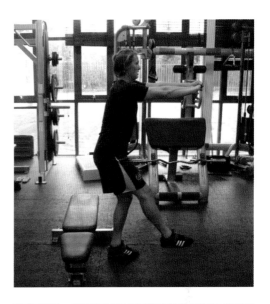

Another screening exercise (single leg squat). As evident, there is a slight amount of knee valgus as the subject goes into flexion, which could be a slight weakness in the hip abductors or a lack of ankle mobility. It is again up to the coach to refer this athlete to the physiotherapist for more thorough examination prior to programme prescription.

Also, with scoring derivatives of FMS, it is imperative that the same person scores athletes and their adaptations and carries out re-testing over time, as the score is based on a scale of 0–3; this minimizes errors and reduces the level of subjectivity within the scores. Depending on what has been noted during assessment, the athlete is then given a second score of weakness, tightness, and/or motor patterning. This would indicate a training focus on particular joints. For example, it may be posterior chain strength and single leg stability work required for knee valgus, mobility programmes for lack of depth or compensation to reach that depth, or motor patterning technical programmes if required. It is essential that these results are put into practice and dictate individual programmes, as these issues have been highlighted as a potential injury concerns. It is important in my opinion that each institute comes up with their own scoring system, which checks for particular things you are interested in, such as

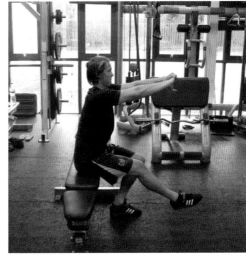

An effective single leg stability exercise. The single leg sit down focuses on the eccentric phase of the single leg squat, controlling the movement as much as possible. It is important that the alignment of the knee remains and the movement can be controlled all the way down. Start with less depth in novice athletes and then increase the depth of squat. Furthermore, the athlete can then increase the load they are lifting.

knee valgus, asymmetrical weight shift, excessive forward lean and so on.

The photographs demonstrate two subjects when performing the overhead squat screening. Both subjects show dysfunctions that need to be addressed. Subject A shows a lack of ankle mobility with possible tight lateral gastrocnemius, forcing the feet to turn outwards when squatting. The lack of ankle mobility causes excessive forward lean. Subject B shows a lack of mobility in the ankles and hips limiting full depth of the squat as well as thoracic mobility limiting the retraction of the scapula.

It is essential that once this test has been done the athlete is then referred to the physiotherapist to perform specific ROM tests at the highlighted joints. Key areas specifically highlighted are the ankle, hip and thoracic spine. This combination of tests will then provide a passive ROM score, as well as how it is integrated into a dynamic movement such as an overhead squat.

Single leg stability

Another test that should be implemented within the screening process is the single leg squat, not to assess for ROM, but to assess the stability properties of the athlete. Ensuring a partial depth without any compensation from the trunk, hips or knees is imperative for the stable athlete. Issues around the athlete's posterior chain to control the knee and hip, as well as their anterior/posterior slings, can be further highlighted in this test. As mentioned in the opening paragraph of this book, mobility and stability are essential for providing the athlete with the potential to become robust, and can be assessed subjectively through the overhead squat and single leg squat exercises. There is much research out there discussing the various issues concerning ROM and single leg stability. The National Association of Sports Medicine (NASM) Corrected Exercise Book, edited by

Clark and Lucett (2010), provides an advanced and detailed approach to corrective exercise.

ROM VS. PERFORMANCE

Although having a greater ROM can be beneficial for performing particular movements required within the gym, and a possible reduction in acute/chronic injuries when training, there are some sports that require lower levels of ROM due to conflicting adaptations. For example, a long distance runner needs high levels of stiffness, especially around the ankle complex as this would optimize the efficiency and utilization of the stretch shortening cycle (SSC), therefore enhancing performance (Dumke et al., 2010). Furthermore, if there's no pain due to high levels of tightness or stiffness, then the practitioner should avoid trying to increase the ROM around the lower limb of an athlete from that particular sport. Many coaches try to increase ROM for these particular athletes to be able to perform certain exercises in the gym, or avoid overload injury due to the athlete's dysfunction. For example, athletes with poor ankle ROM struggle to reach good depth in a squat, and coaches spend a huge chunk of their time trying to increase their ankle mobility to get them to perform a good technical squat, which in turn could possibly reduce the performance level of that athlete. Instead, maintain the high level of stiffness and accommodate this particular type of athlete by putting some plates underneath their heels, providing dorsiflexion so good depth can be achieved whilst they squat, without altering properties that are essential for performance.

It is important to remember the huge benefits endurance runners gain from strength training and squatting, so the exercise should remain a key part of an endurance runner's programme with alterations made, so more posterior chain activation is achieved, providing a greater stability to the knee and reducing the quadriceps:hamstrings ratio.

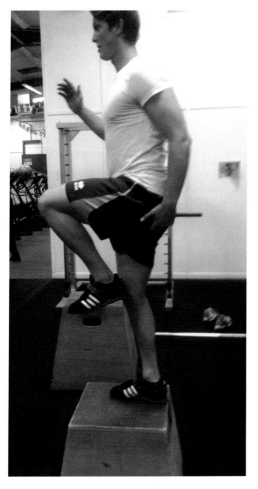 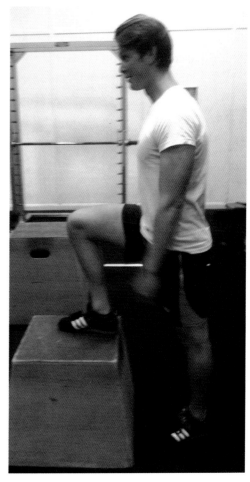

Similar to the single leg sit down exercise, the reverse step-up/step-down exercise focuses on the eccentric phase of the movement controlling the movement as much as possible on the way down. Alignment of the knee is again essential. Increase box height and add load to increase the intensity of this exercise.

Many coaches could argue that it is active stiffness of the musculature required on ground strike that is essential to endurance performance, and that passive stiffness of a structure needs to be reduced. However, I believe that the stiffness/ROM levels will have a transfer, so caution should be taken with endurance athletes. This does not mean that I neglect poor ankle mobility in other sports for performance benefits. However, for this particular sport, unless the stiffness is causing issues or higher injury risk, increasing ankle mobility could be detrimental to the success of that athlete.

With other sports where high levels of ROM are desired as opposed to high stiffness levels, then ankle mobility should be targeted and prioritized. Ankle mobility is often a neglected quality when assessing athletes and needs to be considered in more detail, depending on the athlete and sport.

It is also very important to remember when discussing ROM within squatting is that certain athletes outside of distance running cannot achieve full ROM. Obviously, this needs to be addressed and mobility work should be prescribed to achieve greater ROM at joints that are required. However, coaches should still in the meantime perform strength training in the ROM the athlete does have. It makes sense to get that athlete stronger in the ROM they do have, whilst mobility work is being implemented alongside strength training. Too many coaches will not load the athlete up until they reach a sufficient ROM in the squat. This approach wastes time in getting the athlete stronger and performance benefits may be missed during this period. Remember, the posterior chain can be targeted in other ways if not getting sufficient stimulus and depth from the squatting exercise.

In conclusion, although there is very little evidence around ROM and injury prevention, it is often a quality that is desired within our athletes. If an athlete can possess high levels of mobility at particular joints, it eliminates one reason why they might be getting injured, or might be compensating at another joint, and it enhances a particular biomechanical aspect for the athlete. One thing I have often noticed is that if an athlete lacks range of movement at a particular joint, it might not necessarily be that joint that becomes injured. For example, if an athlete lacks high levels of mobility at the ankle, then issues around the knee could occur, so the practitioner is urged to look at the whole kinetic chain before assuming the cause of the problem. In conjunction with increasing the ROM properties of an athlete, if they can become stable both bilaterally and unilaterally, then the building blocks are set for performance enhancement and injury prevention.

4 A FOCUS ON SHOULDER STABILITY

The majority of the book so far has discussed and favoured the lower limb when discussing injury prevention strategies. The next two chapters will look to enhance strategies to regions above the waist and trunk line when attempting to maximize injury reduction techniques. Having said this, it must be remembered that we cannot simply isolate segments of the body and we need to consider the body as a chain and that every preceding joint movement affects the next. However, finding a breakdown in the chain, or where the movement and force efficiency is reduced, provides a rationale to fixing and enhancing that particular area. Within many sports, the shoulder joint and relevant musculature and connective structures that surround it are essential for performance. This chapter will focus in particular on shoulder stability in various sporting scenarios and how to develop the greatest adaptation, which can transfer to sporting movements effectively. Furthermore, it will look at the caveat of mobility and range of movement at the shoulder following on from the last chapter, and how this quality can assist stability and enhance the overall functionality of the shoulder.

Firstly, it is very important to understand what shoulder stability is. It means ensuring the glenohumeral joint is stabilized during various movements (Bigliani et al., 1996); remember it is a ball and socket joint so has a large ROM with varied directions of movement to control. The aim of increasing shoulder stability would be to reduce any tear or possible impingement occurring to the joint (Weldon and Richardson, 2001), as well as providing an effective base for high force/velocity tasks within certain sporting actions (Siff, 2003). Interestingly, high levels of fatigue acutely decrease shoulder stability and so the shoulder is more vulnerable to injury (Carpenter, Blasier, and Pellizzon, 1998). It must be remembered that many sports require effective shoulder stability, providing a base for high velocity performance in throwing/bowling, racket sports, spiking in volleyball, boating sports and so on. It would also be essential for maximizing stability in high end catching sports such as basketball and goalkeeper positions in soccer. It is therefore an essential physiological skill and adaptation required by many athletes. One very well-known method of enhancing shoulder stability is targeting the muscles and connective structures surrounding the shoulder joint, known as the 'rotator cuff

Rotator Cuff Muscles

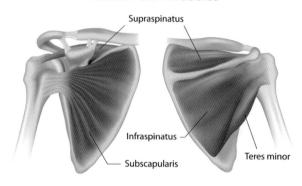

Anterior view   Posterior view

The muscles of the shoulder.

muscles' (Dark, Ginn, and Halaki, 2007). There are four muscles as you can see in the diagram: supraspinatus, infraspinatus, subscapularis, and teres minor.

Each muscle provides and is responsible for different movements around the shoulder joint and therefore can be trained in isolation. For example, the infraspinatus and teres minor aid in the external rotation of the arm, the supraspinatus is the prime mover for the abduction of the arm and the subscapularis internally rotates the humerus. Ways in which these are trained in isolation are demonstrated in various exercises below.

The reason why these potential training exercises are not expanded and discussed in much greater detail is due to my personal opinion on them. It must be noted, firstly, that

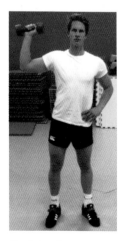 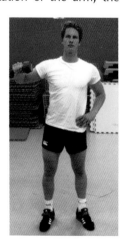 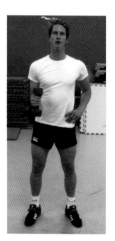 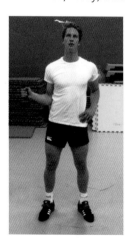

Traditional rotator cuff exercises. It is important that low threshold intensities are used with these exercises, otherwise larger muscles such as the deltoids will be recruited; the aim is to recruit the smaller stabilizing muscles.

effective rotator cuff exercises are incorporated with those that require the effective transmission of forces through the body's kinetic chain. It then becomes more realistic to the forces that are required in the sporting movement, utilizing the force produced from

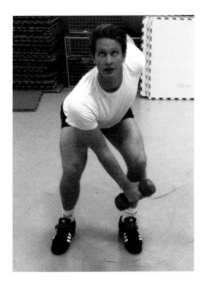

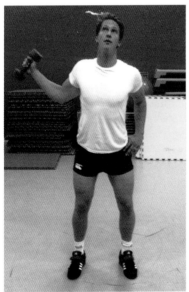

The modified rotator cuff exercise, which utilizes the body's myofascial sling, ensuring the athlete can transfer force through the kinetic chain before stabilizing the movement at the shoulder joint.

the ground. The force is then transferred using the myofascial sling through the body and provides the rotational aspect of the shoulder (McGill, 2009). Creating an effective myofascial sling, and reducing the leakage of energy throughout the trunk will be discussed in much greater detail in the next chapter. The modified exercise therefore, for the rotator cuff exercise, would entail a triple extension with a transfer of force through the trunk and external rotational movement of the shoulder joint. It must be noted that these rotator cuff exercises require extremely low loads, and if heavier ones that are used, the threshold of load will be too high and the movement will be generated through other prime movers such as the deltoids (Dark, Ginn, and Halaki, 2007). Athletes in the gym frequently try to progress the load too high for these types of movements, which in fact becomes counterproductive.

For effective shoulder stability, transferable to the sporting scenario, the whole unit has to be targeted as a whole and strengthened. So isolating a particular rotator cuff muscle would be sub-optimal for creating globalized shoulder stability in a healthy athlete (Burkhead and Rockwood, 1992). In athletes that have injured a particular rotator cuff muscle that needs to be strengthened within the rehab programme, it is essential that this type of exercise is performed. Also, if there is a significant imbalance between internal and external rotators, then an attempt to reduce the deficit is required, by isolating a particular movement. However, if the whole shoulder unit is functional but needs to be progressed, then it needs to be trained as a whole functional unit, not in isolation. The best modalities and exercise prescription for training shoulder stability as a whole would be any overhead exercises (Burkhead and Rockwood, 1992), predominately the overhead squat, as the progression and load that can increase are much greater and will provide greater adaptation (Fleck, 2004). A

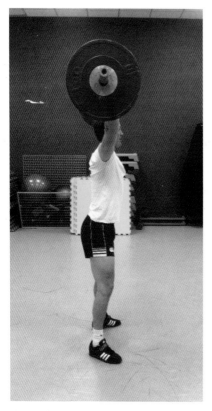

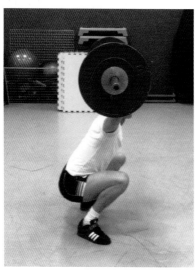

The overhead squat and lunge exercise: a great way to develop shoulder stability through functional dynamic movements.

number of overhead exercises can be done, and to challenge the athlete further, provide the overhead stability tasks with various movements in a variety of different directions and planes, which will add depth to the adaptation. A more novel approach to prescribing a high variety of tasks is encouraged, especially with younger athletes, as it provides a greater range of stimuli for a similar if not the same adaptation (Lloyd and Oliver, 2012).

Another key training modality that can be used to enhance shoulder stability within the prescribed strength programme is unilateral resistance exercises (Prokopy *et al.*, 2008), briefly discussed in Chapter 1 regarding globalized strength training, although bilateral strength will also provide some benefits in shoulder stability. Prescribing unilateral push and pull exercises in both horizontal/vertical force directions would require effective stabilization at the shoulder joint to control the required force production. This helps provide a stimulus where both limbs would be put under stress in isolation, minimizing any imbalance between the two. Once again, variation within the push/pull exercise is optimal for adaptation, placing a novel stress to the shoulder joint when possible. It is up to the individual coach to decide when to apply a new stimulus. This method reinforces the philosophy outlined in this chapter, that shoulder stability exercises should be trained as part of a whole kinetic chain, not in pure isolation, unless an injury rehab rationale requires it.

STABILITY VS. ROM

Creating good shoulder stability through various exercises, some of which are described above, is proposed to be effective in reducing injuries at the shoulder. It is important now to discuss the topic of the last chapter and how as practitioners we can attempt to create the most robust shoulder, enhancing shoulder stability and good mobility as the optimal combination for shoulder health and function (Bak and Magnusson, 1997).

When implementing the overhead squat, it should be a required technical and physical adaptation that an athlete can hold the bar above the crown of the head or even further back for the duration of the exercise (Baechle and Earle, 2000). Although the position of the bar is often debated, when the load is progressed, the greater mobility of the shoulder and position of the bar behind the crown of the head mean that an athlete has a greater chance of stabilizing the movement. If the bar is held too far forward, as soon as the load progresses above a certain threshold the bar will drop forward and will be unable to be maintained throughout the lift. Therefore, it is essential from a technical and structural point of view that within these types of exercises, especially the overhead squat, that a full range of movement from the shoulder is cued. It also important that the shoulders' range and stability should be symmetrical in both limbs, as this has been proposed to be problematic for injury prevention (Bak and Magnusson, 1997). Furthermore, before providing enhanced stability to the shoulder joint, it is essential that the relevant ROM is in place; then stability can be added to it.

THE FUNCTION OF THE SCAPULA

As you can see in the diagram of the shoulder joint, the scapula bone, which attaches the humerus to the clavicle, is clearly visible. In my opinion, the stability and movement of the scapula are amongst the most neglected aspects within shoulder movement and function. Remember, you cannot have strength without stability, and ensuring the scapula and thoracic region of the spine are stable and mobile will underpin a good base

and foundation for the shoulder (Kibler, 1998). The key movements that need to be focused on initially for the scapula, before adding any rotational exercises, are elevation (superior/upwards), depression (inferior/downwards), retraction (adduction) and protraction (abduction). Providing an effective stimulus to ensure these initial movements are able to be completed with no load is essential as a starting point. Exercises such as wall angels, retraction/protraction in a quadrapedal position, and effective elevation and depression in more of a sagittal plane direction are effective. It is extremely important that when the athlete is performing these exercises the strength and conditioning coach ensures that their posture is braced and in a neutral position, and the scapula is being moved in the natural direction, depending on the required movement. Having worked with some very good physiotherapists and sports therapists, interesting observations have been pointed out regarding the natural function and movement of the scapula. Time and experience prescribing these exercises will paint a portrait of what typical efficient movement is in this region.

Once these particular movement patterns are performed well, and an effective platform is set for the movement of the scapula, these exercises can be progressed and loaded, remembering the essential rule of overload for physiological adaptation (Fleck, 2004). Bands can be added to any specific elevation/depression exercise, whilst a reverse fly exercise can be introduced for the retraction and protraction movement, gradually introducing a light load and progressing when able. As well as loading these particular movements, it is now apparent that the function and movement of the scapula can now transfer to the effective pulling exercises such as pull-ups and rows, and pushing exercises such as the bench press. Once the directions of side to side, and up and down essentially have been mastered, focus can be emphasized on any rotational movement of the scapula. With these type of drills such as medicine ball rotations, which serve a primary function of external rotation of the trunk, it is very important that the trunk is stiff and highlights how the kinetic chain is essential not

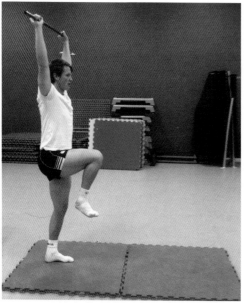

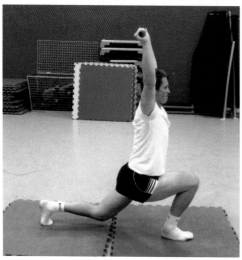

The overhead squat and lunge exercise: a great way to develop shoulder stability through functional dynamic movements.

regions or segments of the body in isolation (McGill, 2009). Once the trunk is braced however, you can observe and coach the movement of the scapula and thoracic region. In my opinion, don't get too wrapped up in what the movement of the scapula looks like in rotational exercise, as it can be very difficult and subjective when observing any dysfunction. What would be important though is the bracing of the trunk allowing the rotational movement and transference of force through the system. This idea will be discussed in great detail in the next chapter and reinforces a clear philosophy that the system as a whole needs to be functional and trained, and a breakdown or glitch in any of the kinetic chain segments could lead to a dysfunction in a particular area. This is when isolation of a particular area is needed. If greater detail or more information is required within the movement of the scapula, and how this underpins effective shoulder stability, the reader is referred to a paper by Kibler; although published in 1998, it has some very good information regarding the scapula.

As a take-home message from this chapter, ensure that the athlete has effective mobility within the shoulder region, which could be underpinned from scapula movement, posture of the shoulder joint itself. After this is established then the athlete can enhance both scapula function and shoulder stability in the techniques provided, before adding strength in that area.

5 | TRUNK STABILITY

For many years the trunk has been identified and established as a key indicator for injury prevention, often termed as 'core strength', although that phrase will not be used in this textbook, as core strength for an aspiring S&C coach would refer to the maximal strength ability in key core exercises performed in the weights room. Instead, the terms 'trunk strength' and 'trunk capacity' will be used. It is widely recognized that the trunk is an essential stabilizer for the body and provides efficiency of movement; although this is true, some methods that have been proposed by various trainers and S&C coaches to enhance this quality are questionable. This chapter will delve closely into the work of Stuart McGill, and his influential textbook, *Ultimate Back Fitness and Performance*. I have had the great pleasure of seeing McGill at conferences and workshops on a number of occasions, and it is my aim to dispel some myths and misconceptions within the area of trunk strength. This chapter will focus on aspects of his work and describe how these can be implemented practically into the strength and conditioning field. First we must identify the aims of the trunk: what we require as athletes and how its strength can be enhanced functionally.

In every sport, effective force transfer is required though the trunk (Brown and McGill, 2009), usually from the force produced from the ground. It is demonstrated that the greater the magnitude of force, the greater stiffness of the trunk required (Brown and McGill, 2008). With running, or any locomotion with effective leg force production and synchronized arm drive, or any throwing event, the aim is to minimize the leakage of energy as it transfers through the trunk region. Even sports such as boxing produce effective punches when high force is generated at the ground, transferred through the trunk and displayed to effective shoulder stabilization and extension of the elbow joint (McGill, 2009). From an injury prevention point of view, the trunk acts as a stabilizer in the middle region of the human body, so a detailed understanding of spine health to avoid injury to such a key area is of the highest priority. The interesting question is, however, how do we train it?

TRAINING THE TRUNK AS A WHOLE FUNCTIONAL UNIT

One common method used for years within therapist/S&C practice and ideology is trying

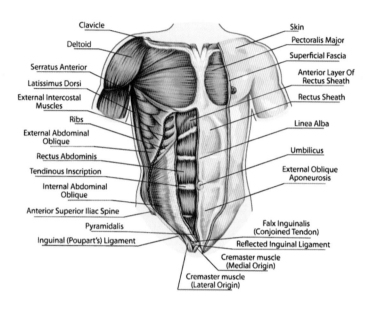

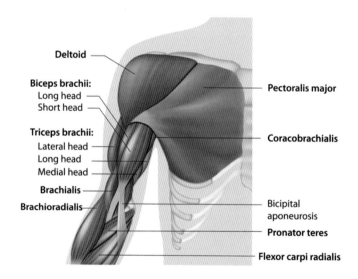

to activate the transversus abdominis (TA) in isolation, and increase the functionality of the trunk. Although this is currently done in stabilizers such as the glutes, it cannot be achieved effectively in the trunk region. It has been used by therapists and in sports such as gymnastics when hollowing has been promoted. This technique is very misleading and contrasting to the desired outcome that we really want within our athletes (McGill, 2009). However, there are always exceptions to the rule, and if an athlete has been sedentary for a period of time due to injury or immobilization within the trunk area, then a brief amount of time initially could be spent on them activating the TA before any extensive rehabilitation work begins (Lee et al., 1998). Within healthy functional athletes, however, this technique should be left alone. Instead, practitioners should focus on training the trunk as a whole functional unit within various different desired movements (Gamble, 2007). This trains the trunk to become effective as a whole unit – otherwise if some muscles are being 'switched on' when others aren't, it could cause imbalance and a lack of efficiency within the trunk.

FLEXION/EXTENSION

Amongst the methods commonly used over the years to enhance the trunk, predominantly in bodybuilding, but also in the sporting environment, are exercises such as sit-ups, crunches and all the variations. Even within well-respected strength and conditioning textbooks (Baechle and Earle, 2000), sit-ups are demonstrated as an abdominal exercise to use. The work of McGill, however, puts forward the risks of this type of repetitive flexion/extension patterns of the spine (McGill et al., 2003), and how they can cause significant damage to spine health. The spine has only a certain amount of tolerance for repetitive flexion/extension patterns before it will potentially 'break'. Common injuries of

this overload of the spine would be a prolapsed disc due to constant overload of sheer forces of the disc between the vertebrae (Parkinson and Callaghan, 2009). Therefore, it is essential that these patterns be avoided within training as athletes will most likely perform them in their sporting movements. If this is combined with poor postural control in everyday life, a percentage of their total spinal vertebrae tolerance will be used up in other activities and adding to this in any S&C training must be avoided (McGill et al., 2003). It also provides a poor training adaptation, and causes the leakage of energy when being transferred through the kinetic chain; this will be discussed in greater detail later.

ACHIEVING A NEUTRAL SPINE POSITION BEFORE ENHANCING STIFFNESS TOLERANCE

Starting with the complete basics of trunk training, an athlete must be able to understand what a neutral spinal position feels like, and to do this a little bit of time must be spent getting the athlete to dissociate extreme movements of the trunk. For example, athletes need to learn the spinal movement from flexion and extension of the lumbar spine under no stress or compression to discs (McGill and Norman, 1987). For example, get an athlete in a quadruped position on the ground with spine position in neutral. Then get the athlete to tuck their pelvis under them to achieve full flexion and then bring their pelvis 'up' and use the glute muscles to create hyperextension of the lumbar spine. You can then get them to identify the range of movement the trunk can go through with full flexion and extension, and activate key musculature in doing so. The most important aspect of this type of exercises is that the athlete can understand how to achieve a neutral spinal position and gain a trunk proprioception of what neutral spine position is, as this will be an essential position for sporting movements/spinal health, and injury prevention.

Once this base of neutral spine has been applied, it is now time to enhance the trunk's ability to maintain neutral posture over a period of time. The idea is to increase the stiffness of the spine/trunk. To begin with, exercises such as the plank are brilliant and should be progressed to a single time of up to 3–5 minutes (McGill, 2009). This may seem excessive and high volume but the trunk needs to be able to maintain this essential neutral position and brace for different types of movement required. After the athlete has established a high tolerance of stiffness/bracing in a static position, some patterns with

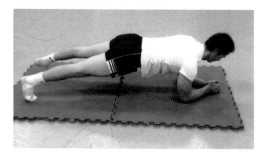

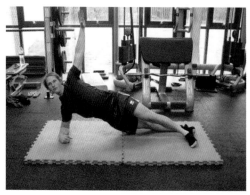

Two plank variations that require neutral spine position to be held over a period of time. These should be the foundations of any athlete's trunk programme.

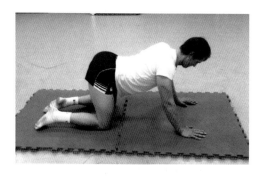

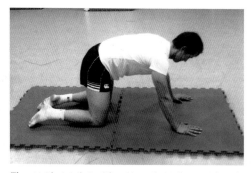

The starting point with any trunk work: ensuring the athlete can move the pelvis appropriately through the ranges, taking the lumbar spine into full extension and flexion. Neutral spine position is in between and should be established by the athlete.

various movements can now be prescribed. However, any movement that is prescribed must challenge the athlete to maintain stiffness whilst moving the arm/leg limbs around the trunk. One of my favourite exercises to demonstrate this is one of Stuart McGill's called the 'stir the pot' (see image below). The Swiss ball has to be 'stirred' in small circular movements, whilst lumbar and trunk remain completely still. Again, build this up to extremely high time durations and tolerance for the spine to be able to hold neutral position, or be stiff for long periods of time. The next stage would to be to add load directly to the static plank – for example, placing some load on the back of the athlete, which puts the trunk under some overloaded strain. The athlete can then progress by

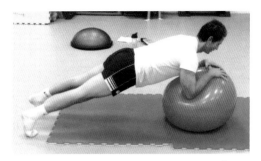

Progressions from the plank are exercises such as 'stir the pot' from McGill, where the trunk is kept stiff whilst the arms rotate in small circles.

increasing tolerance under extra load and so on. This spinal stiffness is essential when first training the trunk, and should be set as a foundation before any rotation or advanced trunk work should take place.

Another indirect way of training the trunk is through the strength sessions being described. Although not the main objective of a session, when lifting in an Olympic lift, squat, or deadlift you can get the athlete to brace externally by getting them to perform a Valsalva manoeuvre prior to the lift, which is a deep breath in and holding it for the duration of the lift. This would then stiffen the trunk during the lift, creating high intra-abdominal pressure and a physiological belt and the required physiological outcome (McGill, Norman and Sharratt, 1990). This study actually looked at applying an actual commercial belt sold for people lifting weights, to keep the trunk stiffer. It was found, however, that when subjects wore this belt a significantly lower intra-abdominal pressure and abdominal activation occurred, providing a poor stimulus and training adaptation for the trunk. Therefore, a lifting belt was not advised. Advice to breathe in on the eccentric phase and out on the concentric phase is no longer recommended for trunk training and the athlete should maintain the breath for the whole repetition. There is caution that this bracing technique causes an acute high blood pressure, but nothing for the healthy athlete to worry about. In fact, in all movements, whether it be a speed/agility task, or in a movement preparation session, athletes should be cued to brace the trunk and get used to keeping it stiff throughout a host of athletic patterns. It should then with good motor learning become autonomous within various sporting movements. A good example of this is ensuring good hip flexion as part of the sprint cycle (high knee drive), with lumbar remaining stable. Hip mobility obviously plays a role in this but stability at the lower back and trunk will also play an essential part.

INTRODUCING TRUNK ROTATION/TRANSFERENCE

Once a foundation has been laid and a high level of stiffness and tolerance has been completed, athletes can now look to enhance their ability in rotation force, or simply training the trunk to be more dynamic. In order to be more efficient within more dynamic tasks, a high level of stiffness has to be present, otherwise any force being transferred will simply be lost or leaked. Within dynamic tasks of the trunk the key is to start with a low velocity exercise, such as a medicine ball rotation and build a good base of movement, ensuring optimal posture is kept for effective transfer of force. Further speed can be developed through the trunk, utilizing our myofascial sling; this means we have a natural way of transferring force due to our anatomical structure, but we have to train this system. The movement cannot simply come from the trunk alone: it has to be generated at the start of the kinetic chain, i.e. the ground, and be transferred through (McGill, 2009). A great example of this would be the shot put, or any throwing event. The force generated in those movements depends on many variables, such as the amount of force that can be generated through the ground initially, but then how much can be maintained and transferred through the kinetic chain without excessive leakage. This means transferring the force through the trunk, which should be braced and stiff and generating high force and velocity in the throwing action. Although it is difficult to train the trunk directly in these type of movements, trunk stiffness is vital, and coaches should focus on maintaining a good, stiff and braced posture with no sign of collapsing. It is therefore the previous stiffness and tolerance work that will have the greatest carry over.

THE IMPORTANCE OF TOLERATING ECCENTRIC LOADING

As well as ensuring athletes can rotate and control anti-rotation effectively, it is essential that they can absorb eccentric loading of the trunk region and maintain good postural integrity. For example, avoiding flexion patterns of the spine but eccentrically loading the trunk region will ensure the trunk is optimally prepared for competition. Exercises such as roll-outs are good for this type of quality, as they eccentrically load the trunk whilst ensuring the spine remains neutral. Note that this type of exercise is very advanced; ensure that the previous stages have been completed first.

Further ways to challenge the trunk

As a strength and conditioning coach, I believe that many useful training modalities are dismissed by those who perceive that lifting is the only way to train. There are often many ways to skin a cat! Training the trunk in this instance can be done in many other ways to supplement the trunk work prescribed within the gym. Exercises such as gymnastic movements and balances on the floor and rings are a great way to enhance stability of the trunk and other areas of the body when trying to complete certain movements and isometric holds. Be creative and challenge the athlete in various movements to stabilize the body effectively.

POSTURAL ASSESSMENT

It is essential when discussing the trunk to mention an athlete's natural posture. It is very difficult to create high levels of stiffness and any other trunk adaptation in training when the athlete defers back to their natural poor posture, particularly with an exaggerated thoracic rounding (a frequent occurrence amongst tall athletes – such as goalkeepers in football and volleyball players – with an extremely long torso). This can be rectified in a number of different ways. Firstly, emphasize to your athletes the importance of standing and sitting up straight. This is unlikely to change the structural properties of your athletes' posture, however, as it is very likely that they have adopted poor habits over time. To combat this structurally, it is essential that the thoracic spine and the mobility of the shoulder is enhanced initially and any tightness in the upper back muscles are eradicated or altered if possible. As well as increasing the mobility, ensuring the scapula movement is functioning well (as discussed in the previous chapter) is essential with creating an efficient trunk.

Athletes with extremely tight pectorals/ latissimus dorsi can have limited thoracic mobility and extension. Once a greater mobility has been identified and sorted, then the real cause of the problem can be addressed, and this issue generally comes down to the posterior chain muscles being really long and weak and the anterior muscles being worked and becoming excessively tight. For example, the pectorals and deltoids might be very tight, due either to genetic structural issues or being worked in the gym at a young age and constantly performing the bench press exercise as a young athlete, with little

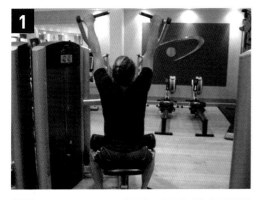
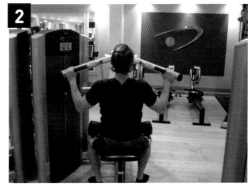
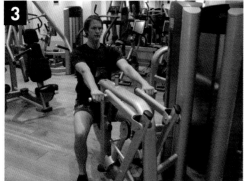
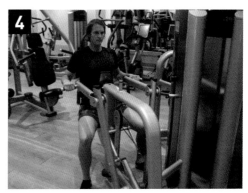

These exercises demonstrate the lats pull down (1 and 2) and seated row (3 and 4), two exercises that isolate the posterior chain muscles (lats/trapezius) and promote effective scapula retraction/protraction.

knowledge of the strength aspect of performance. If over a period of time this is continued, without the relevant counter-balancing of the antagonist muscles, then the anterior working muscles get shorter and tighter, leading to this poor postural model adopted by some athletes. Therefore, it is essential that when gym programmes are prescribed, there is a clear emphasis on pulling exercises being equal to pushing exercises in terms of volumes performed. In my opinion, more volume should be performed on pulling exercises, to create strong posterior chain muscles such as the lower/middle trapezius and rhomboids. For example, when programming, you might prescribe high force work with low repetitions for the bench/shoulder press type exercises, and higher volume with pull-ups/rows. Of course high force and strength is desired in vertical/horizontal pulling exercises, but this should be supplemented with some higher volume pulling work within an athlete's strength and conditioning programme. In fact, although I would not normally advocate any machine-type weights exercise, for postural adaptations such as horizontal/vertical pulling exercises an exception can be made. Exercises such as seated row, or lats pull-down are examples of this. Generally, no machines would be ever recommended in the S&C industry, and the field has moved on past this point, however for a musculoskeletal rationale and isolation of the posterior chain, this type of

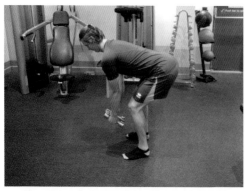 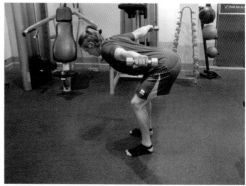

The reverse fly is a good exercise used to enhance the middle trapezius muscles and coincide with the efficient movement of the scapula. The range an athlete can get within the exercise will depend on thoracic mobility.

exercises could be implemented.

In summary, this chapter has explored the importance of avoiding spine flexion within training and certain movements due to the damage it can do to the vertebrae discs. The focus should be upon trying to increase the stiffness of the trunk and maintaining neutral posture for a long period of time, before more ballistic rotational trunk exercises are performed. This not only spares the spine's flexion movement, but also creates an effective training adaptation of transferring force efficiently through the kinetic chain – another clear example of how injury prevention and performance enhancement often go hand in hand. As with shoulder exercises in the previous chapter, particular muscles shouldn't be trained in isolation: the body needs to be trained to work as a functional unit. The exception to this would be within certain rehab periods where certain low threshold exercises could be prescribed, especially focusing on the TA.

Postural awareness has also been discussed, along with the importance of ensuring that the posterior chain is prescribed greater volumes when trying to achieve the optimal posture. For sure, this is not the only way to gain a desired posture – athletes should be given the correct training and mobility work throughout the thoracic spine and at the hips to enable this to occur. Having poor posture (thoracic and lumbar) can lead to several injuries due to lack of mobility and range around those joints. Although there were many references within this chapter, it must be acknowledged that the majority of the research came from Stuart McGill's work within spine health and trunk training. Many of his books on the trunk, which come highly recommended, are listed in the references section.

6 | PROPRIOCEPTION AND PLYOMETRIC PERFORMANCE

This chapter looks at plyometric performance – an important topic that is close to my heart, as the research I have conducted has been in this field. It must be stressed that with efficient training and good programming, plyometrics are not something to be cautious of; if planned correctly, with a progression and continuum set in place for the relevant ability/physical/biological stage of the athlete, plyometrics can demonstrate extremely good gains (Meylan and Malatesta, 2010), and contribute to injury prevention (Myer *et al.*, 2006).

Prior to that, however, and possibly an injury prevention technique in its own right, comes lower level balance work such as proprioception work; this is primarily performed on one leg but can be regressed or targeted bilaterally with different exercises. The main injury prevention aim from this proprioception work would be to increase both ankle and knee stability under a variety of tasks. Aside from the opening chapter on increasing strength, most of the preceding chapters have been about increasing mobility/range of movement at particular joints, whereas now the emphasis is placed on making that range of movement more stable,

in particular in single limb tasks, which could be considered as an essential criterion for injury prevention markers. Although being strong bilaterally has a huge implication on performance and injury prevention, it is essential that an athlete can then transfer this to being strong and stable on one leg, and this chapter will discuss how to do this. Remembering back to the mobility chapter, and how it was assessed in a functional way with athletes, the FMS was proposed (Cook, 2010). Although the FMS looks at the mobility of joints within particular exercises, it also looks at the stability of the shoulder, as previously discussed, and the knee. Therefore, poor stability at the knee/ankle, causing excessive knee valgus or inversion of the ankle would be an undesired trait within our athletes.

LOW LEVEL PROPRIOCEPTION WORK, PREPARATION FOR KNEE STABILITY EXERCISES

As with any modality of training, especially those directly outside of specific sporting skills, it is essential to start from the basics. In an ideal LTAD (long-term athlete development) plan,

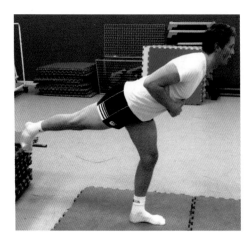
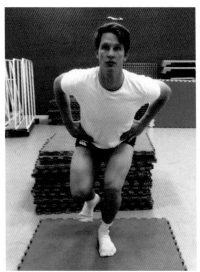

Examples of exercises that provide a good foundation for balance and proprioception qualities. The arabesque exercise is on the left, where it is important to encourage a greater hinge ROM without compensating from any rotation from the hips. The other exercise demonstrates the single leg quarter squat.

this would be done in the introductory years of physical training within academy type structures (dependent on the sport, of course). Please note that the term LTAD here refers to a generalized plan to progress a particular physical quality. It does not refer to the model proposed by Balyi and Hamilton, which will be discussed in much greater detail in the maturing athlete section. Within this period, basics can be implemented, such as an athlete being able to stabilize and balance themselves on one leg for a period of time, then progressing to closing their eyes, or completing other movement competencies such as a catch/throw whilst still balancing. It is also a chance to reinforce the 'athletic position': getting them to balance on one leg in this position, with shoulders over the hips, and knees over the toes. Remember, if an athlete can adopt this position, any multi-directional movement will be easier to perform. This low level single leg balance work provides an effective foundation for ankle/knee stability. A paper produced by McGuine *et al.* (2000) demonstrated that the

athletes who were less competent in the single leg balance tasks were those who experienced significantly more ankle sprains throughout the season, reinforcing the greater ankle stability required for athletes, especially those in sports involving multiple changes of direction. The rationale as to why balance work should be conducted in the athletic position, with slight flexion in the ankle, knee, and hip is that it requires the knee to be stable under flexed position, whereas when all joints are fully extended the vast majority of the stimulus will be placed on the ankle. Furthermore, this encourages the whole kinetic chain to work functionally as a unit. It also enables the athlete to progress to the next stage of this type of work, which is potentially outside the proprioception bracket but fits into a kinaesthetic awareness that it is essential for good stability within athletes. Therefore, ensuring athletes can then control greater flexion on one limb, and control the stability of the ankle and more importantly the knee is an essential adaptation required.

It must be remembered that greater levels

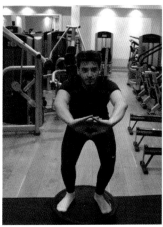 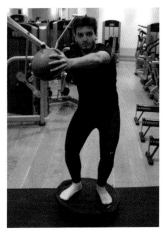 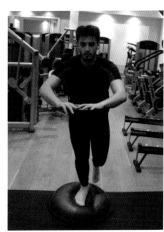

Examples of bilateral/unilateral variations of unstable surface proprioception work. Other tasks such as catching balls of various sizes and weights whilst maintaining good stability can progress this further.

of lower limb strength in these patterns, both bilaterally and unilaterally, will have a great impact on these tasks. However, there are strong athletes that struggle to stabilize the knee in particular movements and this needs to be addressed. Providing a broad set of movements on one limb is proposed to be effective, so the joint/limb is trained to be stable in a range of various movements, ensuring the neuromuscular system is efficient in unpredictable tasks that could occur within sporting movements. Above is an example of single leg control movements that aim to enhance stability at the ankle/knee.

Once these balancing and single leg control movements are performed well on stable environments, the coach can provide an unstable environment on the ground, causing a greater requirement of the proprioceptors and stabilizers to work to control the movement sufficiently. There has been some debate in the past about strengthening on an unstable surface; comical images have been published of someone squatting on a Swiss ball. This is, firstly, very unsafe and secondly, significantly reduces the amount of ground reaction force that can be generated, which is the primal factor in increasing strength. Therefore, the two modalities must be considered as separate, with one maximizing strength and one enhancing stability of the lower limb.

INTRODUCTION TO PLYOMETRICS

When the term 'plyometrics' is initially mentioned, the fear amongst certain S&C coaches, sports scientists and physiotherapists is clear. It must be remembered firstly that athletes, in particular younger athletes, are performing plyometric actions in all sporting activities where they are running and jumping (Ebben and Petushek, 2010) – albeit, these plyometric actions are providing lower levels of stress as contact times on the ground would be considerably higher, unless maximal sprinting is being performed. It must also be noted that when the idea of plyometrics is being introduced to novice athletes, it will be extremely low stress and technical work until they can appropriately increase the stimulus. Therefore, a continuum and progression will be in place, so there should be a competency checklist before athletes can progress on the plyometric spectrum. It is a myth that plyometrics are dangerous; if they are implemented correctly, huge gains can be seen in athletic development and injury reduction. This next section will provide a continuum and progression from low level plyometrics to higher intensity.

Step 1: Promote low level landing

The first stage which follows on from proprioception work, promotes landing mechanics from low heights in a multi-directional approach. The initial phase would teach athletes to land bilaterally off low vertical drops, from horizontal jumps, and jumps in a multi-directional approach. Subsequently, teaching athletes to land correctly in this manner can be integrated into some enjoyable games for effective output and interaction with the athletes. It is assumed that at this stage the chronological age of athletes will be relatively low. However, as discussed previously in the preceding chapters, when an athlete is introduced to strength and conditioning, at whatever chronological age with a low training history, is dependent on factors beyond our control. It is essential that optimal landing mechanics are taught, initially by ensuring the athletes can land softly.

An interesting discussion is occurring in the strength and conditioning field at the moment over the type of coaching cue that is verbally administered to athletes. For example, 'landing quietly' would be an example of an external focus that gives the athlete a task to solve. How they solve it is up to them and could be argued a greater learning tool to develop an optimal strategy for themselves. Another approach would look at giving more internally focused cues that underpin the external focus. Furthermore, to achieve a softer landing the coach could tell the athlete that they need to land on the front of the foot, and then flex the three lower limbs into a squat position in order to dissipate the ground reaction force effectively. This would avoid such high peak forces in shorter time frames

on landing, which has been demonstrated as most likely cause of injury (Jensen and Ebben, 2007; Wallace *et al.*, 2010). Similar biomechanical markers of high forces instantly on ground strike have been evident in running literature as a high source of stress and intensity (Nigg, 1985; Ricard and Veatch, 1994). Ensure a good landing mechanism has been established bilaterally, remembering that there should be good control of the knee ensuring as little valgus (internal rotation) as possible occurs when landing. Furthermore, before progressing to unilateral landing it is important that an athlete can become stiffer on landing and still managing to absorb the eccentric load efficiently, landing in the athletic position as opposed to a full squat position which would potentially spread the impulse over a longer time (Minetti *et al.*, 1998). This would be extremely beneficial for preparing the athletes for further plyometrics and provides them with the ability to absorb eccentric load effectively in shorter time frames, being strong enough to handle that during sporting activity. This adaptation is essential for transfer of injury reduction into the sporting scenario; the athlete will be able to handle eccentric loads on landing and ground strike in high velocity running.

The landing can then be completed unilaterally from a vertical height, or horizontally off the athlete's own jump. Again the progression within single leg landings would ensure the athlete can land softly to begin with, promoting good landing mechanics of holding/maintaining good posture, controlling the alignment of the knee and effective position of the trunk in neutral position. These are all examples of possessing key athletic motor skill competencies (Lloyd and Oliver, 2013). It is very important to understand that enhancing the technical ability to land and stabilize the knee will only cause so much adaptation; if an athlete has severe knee valgus and poor stability further single leg stability and hip strength work will

A bilateral drop jump, where the athlete has landed in an athletic position with high levels of stiffness. This is essential before progressing to single leg lands and on an unstable environment.

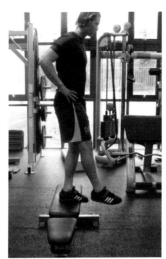
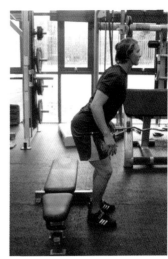

have to be completed to correct this. Also, posterior chain activation and ensuring those muscles are strong enough will also attempt to correct or enhance the stability on one limb. Once an athlete has mastered softer landings on one leg, they can be progressed to generating greater stiffness levels on landing, thus providing a good foundation for plyometric development.

Once low level landing has been completed, further stimulus for the proprioceptors in the ankle/lower limb can be targeted by creating an unstable environment for the athlete to land on. Getting athletes to land efficiently and stabilize the lower limb on an unstable surface, using various techniques and equipment, can see further gains in stabilizing the lower limb in an unorthodox scenario. The proprioceptors therefore have to adapt to control the movement and keep a balanced athletic position on landing. Note that when completing landing tasks in unilateral/bilateral conditions, on stable/unstable surfaces or vertically/horizontally, they should be completed in a multi-directional approach. The majority of sport isn't played through one plane/one direction and although linear work is essential for a starting point, athletes need exposure to

landing in many directions for the exercises to be completely transferable to the sporting situation. It is also advisable to incorporate an element of reactive landing and directions that are unpredictable, to acquire the cognitive skill to control landing reactively (Lloyd and Oliver, 2013). In my opinion, absorbing eccentric load and teaching athletes to land efficiently should be the start of any strength and conditioning coach's plyometric programme, just as deceleration should be the start of any effective agility programme (Hoffman, 2012).

Step 2: Maximize concentric performance

Although athletes perform concentric dominant plyometrics at various different speeds throughout movements in their own sport, it is often done so with very little control. Having completed the preceding phase of landing with single-leg stability and control, the athlete should now have a higher level of control, which can be expressed in higher velocity concentric tasks. Within the landing/control phase some concentric plyometric actions were performed (when executing the horizontal/multi-directional jump and lands, also known as the 'hop and stick'); this phase, however, starts to maximize the gains in concentric dominant plyometrics, increasing explosive power. Coaches are often nervous about providing maximal concentric plyometrics such as high box jumps, especially with younger athletes. However, it must be remembered that when jumping maximally onto a box, the eccentric loading phase, which is considered the most dangerous in terms of load going through the limb, is eradicated, so lower stress is placed on the body in these actions. An unpublished study by Bennett and Goodwin (2011) demonstrated this exactly. The box jump exercise provided lowest peak force, rate of force development and impulse in the first 50m/s due to the landing phase

being eradicated on top of the box.

Prior to suggesting the progressions possible within this stage of plyometric development, it is first essential to understand how enhancing this quality can reduce injury potential. Firstly, it is important to remember that gains can be made structurally, biomechanically and neurologically, especially after the last stage. Due to an enhancement in control and stability of the lower limb, if this can be trained with speed (i.e. higher velocity concentric tasks can be completed with good stability), then ankle and knee injuries that could occur at higher velocities will be reduced. If poor control of the body occurs, especially at higher velocities, repeatedly

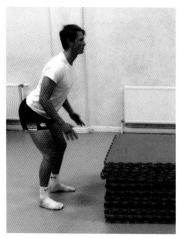
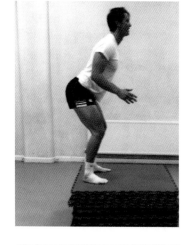
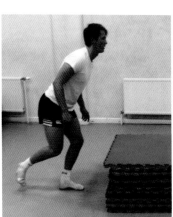
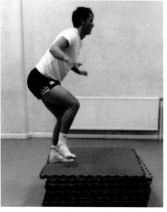

Vertical concentric dominant box jumps performed bilaterally and unilaterally.

within sport, the injury risk will be considerably higher. Therefore, if a biomechanical adjustment can be made and transferred within higher velocity tasks, the potential for injury will be lower.

The second rationale comes from a neurological/physiological point of view, similar to the effects that maximal strength can have on an athlete. If the neuromuscular system can be enhanced, and the body can enhance a greater proportion of motor units within the muscle belly, this can have a greater effect globally within a training programme (Markovic and Mikulic, 2010). For example, the maximal threshold of motor unit activation increases, which then means that the neuromuscular system becomes more efficient when working at sub-maximal levels, the percentage of motor unit activation becomes lower and causes the athlete to be more robust, and therefore can handle greater training loads whilst being less likely to break

down within an overall programme.

Another adaptation that occurs is that the connective structures enable them to transfer force effectively, in particular the Achilles tendon complex (Markovic and Mikulic, 2010). Ensuring the athlete can effectively transfer the high force from the ground and transfer it through the Achilles tendon will ensure that the structure is more tolerable to higher forces within sporting movements. Caution has been advised around tendon overload injuries, and this modality, if not prescribed correctly, could contribute to this overall. However, as noted in Chapter 2, it is essential that the periodization and training programme as a whole is adapted and modified in other areas, so that in plyometric development, adaptation is the primary focus. In Chapter 1 the benefits of maximal strength training were reinforced, but power training and higher velocity actions are also essential for creating a robust, efficient athlete. This is sometimes neglected within the

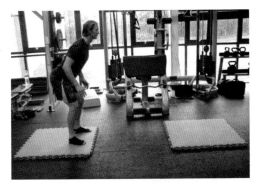
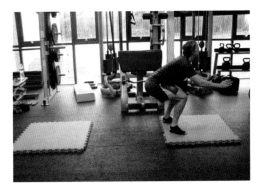
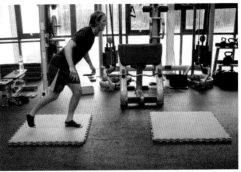
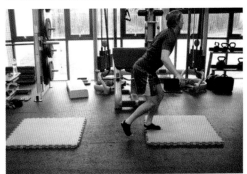

Bilateral/unilateral horizontal jumping exercises, including effective landing control.

S&C, sports science, and physiotherapist fields, and it is simply not enough to create an athlete who moves well: the development of strength and power provides a dimension of robustness, and lower injury levels would result if these physiological qualities were higher in our athletes. A study by Hewett *et al.* (1999) is one of many that demonstrates that plyometric training reduces the incidence of injury, especially within the knee, because it enhances the neuromuscular control to perform that movement.

Step 3: Increase eccentric loading

Once an athlete has developed or enhanced the ability to develop high forces quickly in concentric dominant plyometric exercises, in conjunction with an increase in higher force strength training, they can be placed under higher stress by increasing the eccentric demand. Doing this means they fall off a significantly greater vertical height and are able to control landing. These exercises are often known as altitude drops and were performed in the Eastern Bloc years before they were introduced to the Western world (Siff, 2003). When implementing this aspect of plyometrics, ensure that the number of drops is limited before allowing athletes to progress further (Potach and Chu, 2000).

Once again, progressing the jumps would start with bilateral drops, getting the athletes to land as softly as they can; then, once they can handle dissipating force effectively you can create a higher level of stiffness on landing, providing a solid foundation for the next two plyometric phases. It is essential that an athlete can withstand bilateral drop lands under good control before progressing onto unilateral lands. Minimizing knee valgus and keeping the linearity of the lower limb joints are imperative in reducing injury rates for an athlete on the field. If an athlete can tolerate high eccentric loading both bilaterally and

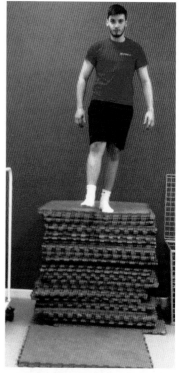

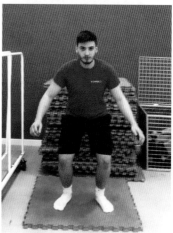

The 'altitude drop', where the athlete is placed on top of a greater height and asked to stabilize the landing. Of course the athlete should be put through the appropriate phases before being prescribed these sorts of exercises. 'Altitude drops' should also be used sparingly and with extremely low volumes due to the high eccentric load on landing.

unilaterally then this will have a significantly positive transfer onto the sporting environment. With higher vertical drops, it is advised that unstable environments are not used, as falling onto an unstable surface could increase the acute injury potential to the lower limb. Unstable surfaces should be kept for use with lower level eccentric landing drills (proprioception balance work) – the athlete needs to control high eccentric loads on a suitably stable surface.

Step 4: Reactive strength development

The next stage in developing plyometric ability is to combine the two stages of plyometric ability together, combining some controlled eccentric load on landing and coupling this with the concentric high velocity phase. It must be remembered that plyometric actions are defined as a rapid lengthening of the musculature (eccentric phase), rapid deceleration of the lengthening phase (amortization), and finally a rapid shortening of the musculature to generate an explosive movement (concentric action) (Ball and Schuur, 2009). Therefore, all of the preceding phases, although not plyometric actions by definition, provide essential foundations and control of the lower limb for completing explosive movements safely in this phase with greater adaptation. Initially, athletes should be coached in singular reactive strength exercises such as the depth jump, where they step off a selected height and try to rebound as high as possible. The natural progression would be to increase the drop height, although when the height increases to where the athlete cannot control the lower limb, and the time spent on the ground is too long, the height should be regressed appropriately. The idea is that the athlete can overcome the eccentric demand on landing as quickly as possible and recoil that elastic energy into an enhanced concentric performance.

This type of exercise can then be progressed to performing jumps in a multitude of directions, and a reactive cognitive element can be introduced too. Furthermore, the exercise can be progressed to single leg depth jumps, ensuring the same short contact time occurs and control of the lower limb is retained. It must be noted that the height of the drop will need to be significantly reduced when performing single leg depth jumps, as

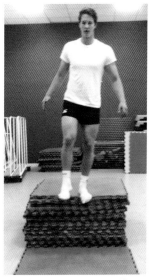

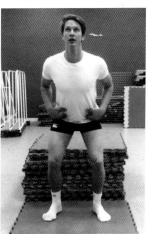

The depth jump exercise where the eccentric/concentric phases are brought together. Encourage greater stiffness on landing as opposed to greater triplr flexion evident in the photo.

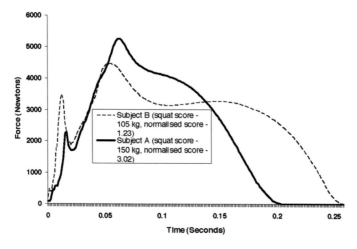

A comparison of force time profiles between two athletes in the depth jump exercise, taken directly from Bennett, Goodwin, and Linthorne (2012).

the same amount of loading will be going through one limb. Biomechanically and physiologically, athletes are looking for a combination of variables to have a significant effect on reducing injuries within their sport.

As evident in the diagram below (taken from an unpublished study by Bennett, Goodwin and Linthorne, 2012) the desired force profile when performing depth jump type exercises would be a lower first peak force on landing, which would indicate that the athlete can deal with the eccentric demands of the task more efficiently, causing lower acute stress to the lower limb. The next two would be potentially performance based: ensuring greater second peak forces and greater impulses in shorter time frames would promote an enhanced concentric performance. In summary, greater plyometric performance would indicate a more efficient and robust athlete who can tolerate greater acute forces and higher training loads as a by-product of increasing power and neuromuscular function. It is interesting to see that the athlete on the graph who had the desired outcomes – such as lower first peak forces, higher second peak forces and shorter ground contact times – had a significantly greater level of maximal strength. This particular study didn't statistically prove that the stronger the athlete was, the greater the

plyometric performance, but it is recommended that an increase in strength will enhance injury prevention/performance in high stress plyometrics. This will be discussed in greater detail in the next section.

Once an athlete has been exposed to this singular reactive strength type exercise, they can be progressed to some higher stress horizontal bounding, both bilaterally and unilaterally. The same criteria apply for these exercises as previously: athletes need to minimize the time they spend on the ground, whilst ensuring lower first peak forces occur, which will significantly reduce injury potential.

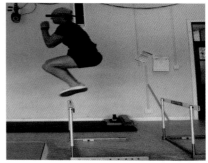

The tuck bound exercise over hurdles, which provides an effective progression from singular reactive strength exercises. Ensuring good control of the lower limb under high velocities and short contacts provides essential injury prevention techniques. Use these exercises well into a programme as the intensity and stress is relatively high.

Once these types of exercises are prescribed, they need to be progressed and adapted again by being performed in all directions and planes to be truly specific to the multi-directional nature of many sports. Note, however, that sports that are linear in nature, such as sprinting, will focus primarily on linear ability, advancing physiological and biomechanical adaptations in that plane and direction.

Asymmetrical jumping performance

It is well established that differences between limbs in any physical quality might lead to a higher injury risk, and jumping performance is no exception. Research (backed up by my own experience) shows that a difference of 10 per cent in jump height ability between limbs would indicate a significant concern for injury. However, it is often advantageous for an athlete to have a more explosive limb, if this is the one that is predominately used within performance. Although both limbs should be efficient within jumping/landing tasks, the coach should not be too concerned if one limb is more dominant and greater at a particular task.

THE IMPORTANCE OF MAXIMAL STRENGTH WITHIN PLYOMETRICS

It has been well documented that an athlete has to be strong to perform plyometrics safely. One of the leading strength and conditioning organizations in the world, the National Strength and Conditioning Association (NSCA) directly suggests that for an athlete to perform high stress plyometrics, they need to be able to back squat 1.5 times their body weight (Baechle and Earle, 2000). Findings in an unpublished study by Bennett, Goodwin and Linthorne (2012) demonstrate that there was no significant correlation between maximal strength scores and performance/injury prevention variables in the higher stress plyometric exercises such as the depth jump. Significant correlations were established, however, between squat score and concentric dominant exercises, such as squat jump and countermovement jump, which reinforces the importance of maximal strength to performance and explains the specificity of the movement and transfer. Nonetheless, although significant results were not established, indirect evidence, comparing the weakest and strongest members of the cohort, demonstrates how maximal strength can impact plyometric performance and injury reduction. However, although I am an ambassador of strength training and believe athletes need to be prescribed a well-structured functional strength programme from as early as possible, the development of eccentric control is compromised by other physical qualities. For example, in the same study, significant correlations were established between lower limb stiffness and first peak force and contact time, providing greater performance and injury reduction potential in those athletes with greater active stiffness on landing. Furthermore, coaches should not refrain from the prescription of plyometric training if an athlete is not maximally strong, as there are other qualities such as teaching athletes to control landing effectively, increasing single leg stability and making them technically more efficient at these exercises, which would elicit greater gains in injury prevention. Coaches should not neglect maximal strength development, however, and more research is needed to assess this hypothesis directly.

BAREFOOT TRAINING

In recent years, predominately within the fields of fitness and health, barefoot training has become a phenomenon that more and more people are using as a tool to reduce injury

(Collier, 2011). Unlike many crazes within this industry, this technique actually has some validity and research behind its application. It has been demonstrated that subjects running barefoot generated significantly lower first peak forces, when running at set velocities and in barefoot conditions (De Wit, De Clercq and Aerts, 2000: Lieberman et al., 2010). This lower first peak impact force (remember from the depth jump diagram that injury potential was attributed to higher first peak force) was demonstrated in the barefoot running condition as the force was spread out over the foot having a flatter surface area on ground strike. Shoes are designed by manufacturers to have substantial heel cushioning, which has altered the natural gait we adopt to a dominant heel-striking stance. This heel-striking stance has led to greater first peak impact forces on ground strike, and could explain potential injuries to repetitive high impact forces when striking the ground during cyclical locomotion. Contrastingly, Giuliani et al. (2011) demonstrated that when subjects wore the newly designed barefoot simulation shoes, and completed the exact same running volume and intensity as previously performed in training, two subjects suffered metatarsal stress fractures along the diaphysis of the foot. Therefore, if someone were to switch to using barefoot style shoes, their running style would have to be adapted from a heel strike to more of a mid-foot strike stance.

The aim of this discussion is not to encourage all of our athletes to start competing barefoot, as this would be disadvantageous to performance, and potentially cause greater injuries, but to consider some barefoot training within the S&C aspects. Furthermore, when prescribing stability work, specific balance work or even fundamental movement pattern work, suggest to your athletes that they perform it barefoot. Although research around barefoot conditions within single leg stability work and so on has not been explored, it will provide a different stimulus to the proprioceptors and require a higher level of kinaesthetic awareness from the athlete. It will also allow the athlete to reach the full mobility within certain tasks, without the aid of particular footwear. For example, greater depth in the squat will be possible, as the heel is already elevated, requiring less mobility from the ankle. Therefore, the true ankle mobility will be tested in barefoot conditions. From a safety and performance enhancement point of view, any heavier strength and power development should be performed in shoes that the athlete feels comfortable wearing and can elicit greater results. From a plyometric point of view, too much of a cushioned heel would take away the forefoot ground contact that is required, which enables the S&C coach or sports scientist to make a personal judgement on the information they have. Any readers who are particularly interested in barefoot running, and the possible benefits and limitations associated with it, are recommended to read an interesting review by Jenkins and Cauthon (2011).

To summarize this chapter, a clear progression of introducing proprioception/balance work through to high stress plyometric training has been issued. If coaches can produce athletes who are stable on one limb, especially at the knee and ankle joints, the starting point for plyometric training becomes apparent. Then a combination of effective landing mechanics, transferring that stability to higher eccentric load tasks, and progressing to being able to express force fast and efficiently, the ultimate robust athlete will be created. Of course, there are many variables that can account for an athlete's injury, and as experts in the field we need to try to eradicate any issue that could potentially cause injury. Although this section only focuses on one aspect of injury prevention, I strongly believe that it is one of huge importance and athletes should be exposed to higher stress plyometric exercises to progress further. Continuing lower level balance and eccentric load work alone may not be sufficient in preparing an athlete for the demands of their sport.

7 | THE FEMALE ATHLETE

The next two chapters explore how injury incidence can be reduced within a particular population; here we discuss the female athlete, the considerations that have to be taken into account, and how to modify training programmes appropriately. The anatomical and structural differences are explored, and also hormonal or historical issues that might affect physiological and physical qualities relating not only to injury potential, but also to health and well-being. It must be remembered that as coaches, we are looking to adopt a holistic approach in providing an optimal support service to developing athletes. Although as S&C coaches injury prevention within any athlete is a high priority, the overall well-being of athletes is essential. What will be also reinforced throughout this chapter is the fact that many of the points discussed (although obviously not all) may be relevant to male athletes. Many of the techniques and training modalities used can be applied across the board, and may have already been suggested in preceding chapters for a host of reasons.

GREATER RISK OF INJURY

It is well documented that within sports that have higher elements of jumping and change of direction, females have a significantly greater incidence of injury – a four- to six-fold increase (Arendt and Dick, 1995). According to NCAA statistics, more than one in ten females demonstrate injuries to the knee (Hutchinson and Ireland, 1995). Injuries to the ACL (anterior cruciate ligament) are generally the most common – due, it is believed, to the greater Q angle in females (the angle of the femur to the knee and then from the knee to the hip at the respective attachment points) (Horton and Hall, 1989). The Q angle is shown in the diagram below. The anatomical structure of the female pelvis is considerably wider, this width and stability being necessary in childbirth. It does however, propose a problem for control of the knee within various movements, and explains the higher injury rates. A greater internal rotation of the knee is therefore more evident, the knee moving inwards when performing certain movements. This is known as knee valgus and is a precursor for injury rates to the ACL. There are three main injury prevention techniques that should be implemented. Firstly, it is essential

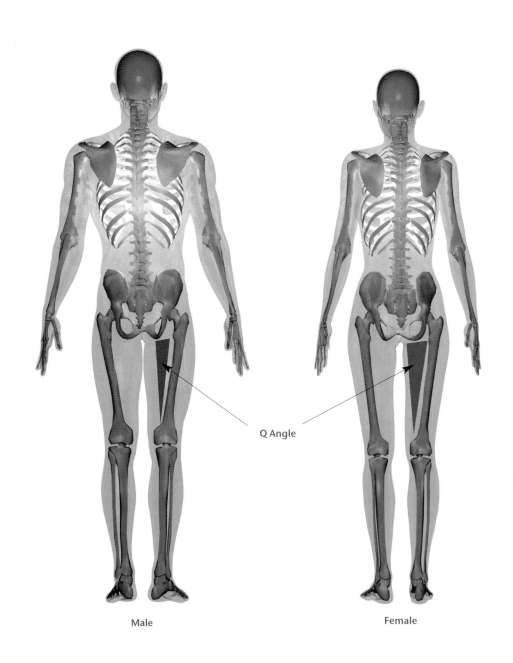

Male

Female

Q Angle

The difference in Q angles between male and female.

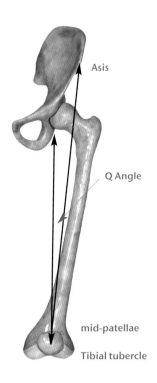

Asis

Q Angle

mid-patellae

Tibial tubercle

The Q angle.

the posterior chain have been previously discussed; however, it is an essential training tool within the female population. Firstly looking at the hamstrings group of muscles, and attempting to reduce the quadriceps:hamstring strength ratio in female in athletes is essential. Strengthening the group of hamstring muscles has been demonstrated to reduce injury rates at the knee significantly (Croisier *et al.*, 2008), mainly due to the function the hamstrings play in stabilizing the movement and alignment of the knee joint (Olsen *et al.*, 2005). Although exercises such as the hamstring curl are effective at loading the hamstring and strengthening it (Baechle and Earle, 2000), coaches are urged to increase hamstring strength during lengthened states. For example, exercises that require the eccentric phase of the exercise to be under load are preferable when strengthening the hamstrings. Exercises such as the Nordic exercise can be implemented at very early chronological/training ages, ensuring athletes can control their bodyweight initially. Then coaches can prescribe higher load type exercises such as RDLs or 'good mornings', etc. To ensure athletes are technically efficient at exercises such as these, it is essential that they are taught to hip hinge from an early age under no load, so they can dissociate the movement from the hip away from other exercises such as squatting that are knee-dominant. Once athletes are technically able to perform both exercises, it is important that both of them are incorporated into the programme.

that the posterior chain is worked on, the glutes and hamstrings specifically. Secondly, focus on landing and deceleration mechanics, progressing onto a well-structured plyometrics and agility programme providing the required neuromuscular adaptations. Lastly, ensuring good mobility and stability of joints either side of the knee can significantly enhance the stability of the knee. These three points will be discussed in greater detail in the next section of this chapter.

INCREASING POSTERIOR CHAIN STRENGTH

One way of attempting to reduce occurrence of knee injuries in females is to strengthen the posterior chain. Exercises and ways to enhance

Furthermore, the hamstrings are a bi-articular muscle (Van Ingen Schenau, Bobbert and Rozendal, 1987), which means it crosses over at two joints. It is then responsible for extension of the hip, and flexion of the knee so both exercises are required to train the hamstrings at either end of hamstring range. Therefore, training the hamstring under eccentric hip extension (RDL/good morning) and knee flexion (Nordic) would provide the optimal strengthening of the hamstrings throughout the whole range.

The gluteal muscles also play an important role in controlling the alignment of the knee effectively. Focusing on glute max initially with exercises such as deep squatting (Caterisano *et al.*, 2002), unilateral exercises such as lunges (Bodreau *et al.*, 2005), and glute bridges all provide an essential stimulus to that muscle. It is important also that glute med/min are targeted as well, with the use of the hip abduction bodyweight/band exercises. A complete glute prehab session was provided in Chapter 1. Enhancing the athlete's ability to activate and strengthen the glutes is essential for reducing lower back pain, and overload of the hip flexors. If an athlete cannot switch on the glutes when required, every movement they do will be performed and compensated either by the hamstrings, and lower back muscles, or the hip flexors. The aim is to enhance the endurance within these prehab exercises, as this will strengthen the glutes over a larger volume of low threshold work and would transfer to controlling the alignment of the knee throughout the exercise period. The high force, low volume strengthening should also be completed with maximal squatting and heavier single leg exercises. It is important to note that increasing the maximal strength of the glutes will also indirectly enhance their endurance capabilities. The increase in the efficiency of the muscle working at sub-maximal intensities is due to increasing the maximal number of motor units that can be activated (Siff, 2003). Nonetheless, specific glute endurance work should be prescribed within prehab modalities.

It is therefore essential that for female athletes, the posterior chain (hamstrings/ glutes) is strengthened significantly and a high percentage of the S&C programme is required to ensure the athlete remains injury-free. The outcome will potentially reduce the ratio between quadriceps and hamstrings, and control the alignment of the knee, which in turn will reduce knee injuries – ACL injuries in particular. As well as enhancing the posterior chain, other neuromuscular training programmes can also enhance the stability of the knee, and should supplement posterior chain strengthening.

NEUROMUSCULAR TRAINING

It is proposed that the majority of knee injuries occur during jumping/landing and change of direction activities. Therefore, to accommodate and complement posterior chain strengthening, it is essential that a neuromuscular training programme is prescribed within these motor skills/patterns. Coaches should initially work on effective landing mechanics within vertical/horizontal drops, as well as deceleration mechanics prior to any high velocity jumping and change of direction. Once these skills have been developed, then the athlete can complete a more advanced plyometric and agility programme. A complete stage progression of a plyometric training programme has been outlined in Chapter 6. Two studies by Hewett *et al.* (1996a; 1996b), demonstrate that an effective plyometric programme can reduce the number of ACL injuries within female athletes by 50 per cent. However, the injury rates were still 2.4 times greater than amongst men, reinforcing the importance of trying to reduce ACL injuries within females. Myer *et al.* (2006), demonstrated that both plyometric and balance programmes significantly reduced the incidence of ACL injuries in females, and should both be an integral part of a female's strength and conditioning programme. Lastly, Mandelbaum *et al.* (2005) provide further statistical information that an integrated balance, plyometric and agility programme showed significant decreases in ACL injuries in females, and reinforces the importance of all of these neuromuscular and

Reference	Design	Average PEDro Score[*]	Population	Intervention	Frequency	Duration, min	Instructional Training
Hewett et al[2]	Prospective, non-randomized, cohort study	4	High school female soccer and basketball players	Three-phase program included flexibility, plyometrics, and weight training, with emphasis on technique, strength, power, agility, and performance	Three alternating d/wk, 6 wk before start of season	60 to 90	Certified athletic trainer and physical therapist demonstration of stretching and plyometric techniques with emphasis on proper form and coach and certified athletic trainer feedback regarding technique
Myklebust et al[9]	Prospective, non-randomized, crossover study	4	Elite Norwegian female handball players	Five-phase program with 3 exercises (floor, balance mat, and wobble board)	Before practice, 3 d/wk for the first 5 to 7 wk, then 1×/wk for the remainder of the season	15	Instructional video and posters with physical therapist feedback regarding technique
Mandelbaum et al[13]	Prospective, non-randomized, cohort study	5	Female soccer players, aged 14 to 18 y	Warm-up, stretching, strengthening, plyometrics, sport-specific agility drills	Before practice, 3×/wk	20	Instructional video and supplemental literature with emphasis on proper technique
Petersen et al[10]	Prospective, matched cohort study	4	Elite German female handball players	Six-phase balance board and jump training program	Before practice, 3×/wk in preseason, then 1×/wk for the season	10	Video and educational session regarding mechanism of anterior cruciate ligament injuries
Olsen et al[7]	Prospective, cluster randomized control trial	7	Female handball players, aged 15 to 17 y	Exercises with a ball, wobble board, and balance mat were used for warm-up, technique, balance, and strength/power	Before practice at every training session for first 15 sessions, then 1×/wk for the remainder of the season	15 to 20	Exercise books and single visit from an instructor from Handball Federation to improve awareness and control of knees and ankles

[*]PEDro indicates Physiotherapy Evidence Database.

Hewett *et al.* demonstrated that a plyometric programme can reduce the number of ACL injuries among female athletes.

proprioception aspects within a female's strength and conditioning programme.

There is a huge body of scientific evidence regarding exercises that will increase the alignment and control of the knee in female athletes, but how the programme is constructed and coached by the practitioner is essential. Correct technique and progression is essential for the content to have significant impact on ACL injuries and knee function. Also bear in mind that a plyometric/agility programme alone is not enough to minimize the effect of ACL injuries, and coaches should remember the importance of increasing the strength of the lower limb, especially the posterior chain as discussed earlier. Another important aspect of knee-injury reduction is ensuring good movement and control of the joints above and below the knee joint, which will be discussed in greater detail in the next section of this chapter. Furthermore, the practitioner should also be aware that plyometric and agility programmes should be prescribed firstly in a linear way under predictable conditions so the athlete can gauge a kinaesthetic awareness of the movement with good neuromuscular control. It then has to be prescribed under multi-directional and unpredictable conditions, as this is what will occur within their sporting environment.

IMPACT OF THE HIP AND ANKLE JOINTS

This next theory of how to enhance the stability of the knee is one that derives from the joint-by-joint approach advocated by Gray Cook and Michael Boyle, two popular S&C coaches in America whose views (often differing from UKSCA recommendations) favour a more movement-based approach over a high loading philosophy. Personally, I seem to sit in the middle of the two, as strength training is an essential aspect of the physical profile of an athlete, as is good mobility. Cook's approach looks at the body in more of a global sense and understands that the body is like a chain, not isolated joints acting on their own. Therefore, if we see poor stability at the knee, the cause could be at either the joint above or below that – the ankle or the hip joint. My own experience backs this up: a weakness at the knee can be seen at either the joint above or below. For example, a significant lack of ROM at the ankle or hip, and a possible lack of stability at the ankle can then demonstrate issues around the knee. Common outcomes of a lack of ankle ROM within an athlete are high levels of knee valgus. Therefore, it is essential that a coach looks at this information when attempting to rectify the issue. It can be easy to target direct issues that relate to the knee, like posterior chain strength, or other neuromuscular training modalities, but as scientists we have to assess the body as a kinetic chain, and look at all of the joints. Furthermore, there might be another issue affecting the knee that has been overlooked, and the coach is urged to assess the athlete in greater detail, and attempt to fix the problem as best as possible.

THE FEMALE ATHLETE TRIAD

This next section concerns an issue that derives from a combination of psychological and physiological factors, the Female Athlete Triad

(Nattiv *et al.*, 2007), that is to say the relationship between a low energy intake, low bone mineral density (BMD), and menstrual dysfunction. Each aspect of the triad will be discussed in greater detail in the next sections, but it must be noted here that a low energy intake, low BMD, and a dysfunctional menstrual cycle (known as amenorrhoea) lead to a significant reduction in performance and health. (Note that for financial reasons, in many clubs/organizations your role may not be limited to just S&C, and knowledge of other concerns and duties will be an essential in both elite and non-elite environments. This reinforces the importance of a holistic approach to sports science support and close integration between all areas of expertise.)

Energy availability

As mentioned earlier, low energy intake isn't restricted to just the female population; there is a lack of research within the male population, but it is still evident. Much research is evident within the female population and low energy intakes, however.

Energy availability is defined as dietary energy intake minus energy expenditure (Nattiv *et al.*, 2007). Low energy intakes within female athletes, either with or without eating disorders, can have a significant effect on the physiological function of the body. If energy availability is too low, physiological mechanisms reduce the energy used for important functions such as growth, reproduction and cellular maintenance (Wade, Schneider, and Li, 1996). This compensation tends to restore energy balance and promotes survival but reduces health and well-being in an athlete. Many instances of low energy availability are derived from disordered eating, seen in abnormal eating habits such as fasting, purging, extreme weight loss pills, and binge eating (American Psychiatric Association, 2000). Common disorders include anorexia nervosa and bulimia nervosa. Lack of energy availability is not always achieved by a lack of intake, but a deliberate increase in energy expenditure. Again, this is termed as a form of disorder, and should be treated seriously.

The psychological effects of a low energy availability have been proposed to be closely linked to low self-esteem, depression and anxiety disorders (Rome *et al.*, 2003). However, it must be clear that these other consequences will not always be a direct result of low energy availability, in fact one of these issues could trigger an eating disorder and work in reverse. Caution must be applied when trying to assess the cause, if this is ever presented within your working environment. A number of chronic medical complications are caused by a low energy availability (Becker *et al.*, 1999), not to mention the acute effects of decreasing performance, a reduction in recovery rate, and increase in injury potential. It is therefore essential that it is avoided in the first place, or if it does occur professional help is sought by a psychologist to rectify the problem as quickly as possible.

As daily practitioners, however, we can make a real attempt to avoid any trigger of a low energy availability, with or without an eating disorder. When discussing any body fat percentage results, the terminology and how it is worded by the practitioner should be addressed with extreme care. Professional dietary and nutrition advice should be given on matching the intake with the expenditure, and clear education from a young age should focus on getting the right amount of macro and micro nutrients. Something that can be done within many clubs and organizations to avoid a potential disorder is to avoid publicly revealing test results. What has been evident in many clubs I have worked at, is a list visible to everyone on the board, with the lowest to highest body fat percentage. This, for most people, would be fine and wouldn't affect their psychological state. However, it could cause some form of disordered behaviour in many individuals so should be avoided. A low

energy availability obviously has an impact on the other two elements of the female triad: BMD and menstrual function (Anne *et al.*, 2003).

Bone mineral density

BMD ranges from complete healthy bone to diseases such as osteoporosis. Osteoporosis is simply a lack of bone strength due to a skeletal disorder, increasing the risk of fracture (National Institutes of Health Consensus Development Panel, 2001). Bone strength and fracture risk is said to be dependent on density, the internal structure of bone mineral and the quality of bone protein, which is why BMD isn't always the only determinant in a fracture (Nattiv *et al.*, 2007). However, BMD is proposed to be the biggest factor in bone strength and the one most commonly screened. BMD causes are strongly linked to energy intake, and is caused by either a rapid accelerated bone mineral loss in adulthood, or not accumulating optimal BMD in childhood and adolescence (National Institutes of Health Consensus Development Panel, 2001). Although a lack of essential nutrients such as calcium and vitamin D have a major role to play in this, the knowledge of increasing bone strength throughout childhood through loading and exercises should be remembered: weight bearing exercises such as strength training provide increases in BMD (Hind and Burrows, 2007). It is therefore essential that a well-designed strength programme alongside nutritional intake is administered for optimal BMD. Any disordered activity previously spoken about would therefore hinder the development of BMD, and demonstrates the clear link between the aspects of the Female Triad. BMD can also be affected by the menstrual function.

Menstrual function

'Normal' menstrual function follows a cycle of

approximately 28 days, and consists of different phases within this (Nattiv et al., 2007). The 'normal' or 'regular' menstrual cycle will be discussed later in this chapter; however, this section will focus on the abnormal cycle and its causes and effects on an athlete's health. The regular period cycle lasting approximately 28 days is known as menorrhoea, a cycle that lasts longer than 35 days is known as oligomenorrhoea, and one that is known as the most drastic which lasts longer than 90 days, or three months, is known as amenorrhoea (American Society of Reproductive Medicine Practice Committee, 2004; Vollman, 1977). Amenorrhoea that exists before menarche (the onset of the menstrual cycle in puberty) is called primary amenorrhoea, whereas amenorrhoea that occurs after menarche is termed secondary amenorrhoea (American Society of Reproductive Medicine Practice Committee, 2004). Initial research conducted within animals proposes that an energy deficiency causes delayed sexual development, suppressed growth and development and therefore delayed menarche (Schneider and Wade, 2000). Although many studies are inherently biased, it is suggested that athletes reach menarche at a later stage than non-athletes (Stager, Wigglesworth, and Hatler, 1990). Warren (1980) found that in ballet dancers, menarche occurred at a later chronological age, and at the same height and weight in non-dancers. However, the study would have been more accurate if biological age had been measured, although the study was conducted over 30 years ago and the concept of 'biological' age would have been in its infancy. Furthermore, the later onset of menarche could have been attributed to a poor dietary intake in conjunction with high volumes of physical training. Although studies have failed to identify whether it is physical training alone that can cause a delay in menarche, it is essential that coaches enforce a 'healthy' diet with enough energy intake so a healthy menarche function occurs. It does beg the question whether as coaches we are suppressing females' maturation and growth quality by prescribing forms of physical exercise.

Within experiments conducted on animals, reducing energy intake by 30 per cent or more consistently caused infertility (McShane and Wise, 1996) as well as skeletal demineralization (Mosekilde et al., 1999), reinforcing again the strong link between all elements on the Athlete Female Triad. In the Triad, menstrual disorders result from a lack of luteinizing hormones (LH) secreted from the pituitary gland at the optimal frequency (Laughlin and Yen, 1996). Research confirms that the LH pulsatility is disrupted with five days of a reduction in energy availability in young women by more than 33 per cent, to less than 30 kcal/kg (Loucks and Thuma, 2003). Remember that energy availability is defined as energy intake minus expenditure. If the reader is interested in the science behind how a lack of energy availability can affect LH pulsatility and menstrual function, they are guided to these articles: Filicori et al., 1995; Wade and Jones, 2004; Wade and Schneider, 1996.

Research has shown that amenorrhoea could be induced by increasing energy expenditure through exercises with no alteration of energy intake (Williams et al., 2001a). Ovulation was then restored by increasing energy intake and not altering energy expenditure or training (Williams et al., 2001b). This latter type of amenorrhoea is called functional hypothalamic amenorrhoea. This provides essential information to strength and conditioning coaches: when a greater volume of training stimulus is required for overload, it is essential that energy intake is increased to match the increase of expenditure. This concept may seem simple, but can be easily forgotten.

The Female Athlete Triad: A summary

Although the above section explained the different sections of the Female Athlete Triad in a degree of detail, it is essential to understand the key take-home messages that strength and conditioning coaches should implement in their daily practice. For a female athlete, whatever her age, energy availability should be optimal. The importance of ensuring that energy intake is high enough for daily function, and for the energy expenditure requirements of their sport and training, cannot be stressed enough. Coaches need to also consider the way in which they talk about body composition, and how they publish test results, as a trigger for eating disorders could occur. The effects of a low energy availability on bone strength and function has been demonstrated, as well as the menstrual function. Low level of energy intake will decrease BMD, increasing the likelihood of fractures and injury, as well as causing the onset of menstrual disorders. It cannot be stressed enough that the holistic approach to wellbeing and health is essential for us as coaches, and more consideration needs to be taken of the athlete's lifestyle, not just performance within their sport. Clearly, a significant lack of energy availability will decrease performance, cause greater levels of fatigue and will increase the likelihood of injury occurrence acutely.

THE FEMALE MENSTRUAL CYCLE

Aside from the Female Triad, and focusing on the dysfunction of the menstrual cycle, it is important that the 'normal' cycle is discussed, as this is an obvious difference between coaching males and females and could potentially affect training and injury occurrence.

The menstrual cycle consists of three different main phases. The first phase, which consists of a gradual increase in oestrogen for approximately 7–10 days, is known as the follicular phase. Following this comes the ovulation phase, where an ovum or egg is released from the ovary. If the egg is not impregnated then the cycle enters the last phase, known as the luteal phase. The luteal phase lasts approximately two weeks and sees a significant reduction in oestrogen levels. Within this phase is the menstruation, where bleeding and, commonly, stomach cramps occur in the female. This particular discomfort for females can last anything between three and seven days. Aside from the physical discomfort females are going through at this time (and I urge coaches to know and track the menstrual cycle of their athletes), the important question to ask is: are there stages of the cycle that can have a potential impact on their performance?

Effects on strength/explosive performance

It is known that increasing amounts of testosterone can enhance strength levels significantly; is it logical therefore to ask the question: how do fluctuating levels of oestrogen, which occur so drastically within the female menstrual cycle, affect performance levels? Greeves et al. (1997) demonstrated that when oestrogen levels within subjects were altered, there was no change in muscle strength or fatigability, despite previous claims. However, earlier research by Sarwar, Niclos and Rutherford (1996) demonstrated that within the menstrual cycle phase, there was a significant change in strength and fatigability. Specifically, at mid-cycle where ovulation occurs and there is a significant increase in oestrogen levels, there was an 11 per cent increase in hand grip and quadriceps strength reported. Also identified at this particular phase was an increase in the fatigability of these strength measures and a slowing of relaxation of muscles. It has also been proposed that testosterone levels increase during ovulation, which may be the reason behind an increase in strength levels. This provides important information that strength/power/speed programmes should include high force phases around mid-cycle, with considerably lower volumes, which could cause greater fatigue and enhance the risk of injury. This displays an excellent example of not only individualizing programmes for a required gender, but each individual, when this aspect of the cycle is occurring. What is also evident from the same study, is that for those who were taking the contraceptive pill, which can alter the menstrual cycle into predictable timing or eradicate it altogether, there was no increase in strength or fatigue levels throughout the cycle. Therefore, with athletes using the contraceptive pill, or any other contraceptive method, there seems to be very little fluctuation in sexual steroid hormones, and this could allow the strength and conditioning coach to prescribe training methods without the influence of the menstrual cycle.

Effects on aerobic performance

Despite a significant reduction of fatigue levels in the quadriceps (Sarwar, Niclos and Rutherford, 1996) and respiratory muscles (Chen and Tang, 1989) during the luteal phase, Lebrun *et al.* (1994) demonstrated a significant reduction in aerobic performance in the luteal phase. It was proposed that both relative and absolute VO2 max was lower in the luteal phase in comparison to the follicular phase. This proposes a trade-off for the strength and conditioning coach, in that female athletes would tolerate greater volumes of training within the luteal phase of the menstrual cycle, although the aerobic performance will be lower. Nevertheless, it gives a clear indication that central adaptations

such as maximizing VO2 max would be better off being completed in the follicular phase, whereas peripheral adaptations such as the extraction of oxygen from the blood to the muscle, where low intensities and higher volumes are necessary would be better administered in the luteal phase. This all demonstrates that a high level of detail is required in planning individualized programmes for greater performance gains and reduction in injuries. The coach also needs to consider the effects of concurrent training, and how adaptations of other physical qualities might therefore be interfering with each other.

Effects on spatial ability and cognitive function

As well as the various physiological components that make up sporting performance, spatial and cognitive aspects are equally as essential for particular sports. Examples such as locating the quickest way around the sporting arena, decision-making and kinaesthetic awareness, occur within every sport in different ways. There have been well-documented differences in spatial and cognitive abilities between genders (Kimura, 1992); moreover, Hausmann *et al.* (2000) have demonstrated that there was a significant reduction in spatial ability during the mid-luteal phase in comparison to the follicular. Again, this has been attributed to a decrease in sexual steroid hormones such as testosterone and an increase in levels of estradiol within the body. This suggests that extra caution is needed within sports that require high levels of spatial ability for safety, such as gymnastics, diving and so on; not only could performance be impaired during this time period, but also an increase in injury could occur within these complex sports. A change in programming might be beneficial, where the most complex sequences within this sport could potentially be attempted in the follicular phase, where spatial ability is at its highest (not only for an increase in performance, but also a reduction in potential injury). Competition, however, is not selected by athletes and their support staff, and these dates are out of anybody's control. The use of the contraceptive pill, however, will control the cycle, leaving the athlete in an optimal state for competition, although it must be the athlete's decision whether they want to administer it. A whole host of reasons – including the possible side effects and religious beliefs – might restrict its use; conversely it could provide an opportunity to increase the complexity of cognitive stimuli during training when this phase occurs, in an attempt to keep decision making/reaction levels as high as possible when competing.

EFFECTS OF PREGNANCY

There is a chance that you may work with an athlete who falls pregnant; this section discusses some changes that might be considered during this time to maximize performance and protect long-term performance losses. When an athlete is pregnant, there is no harm in strenuous exercise, if the athlete is already used to that level of intensity. In fact, exercise until late pregnancy has been proposed to have health benefits for the athlete and baby (Artal and O'Toole, 2003). During pregnancy however, some changes occur which coaches need to be aware of. As with the menstrual cycle, there is a change in hormonal release. Throughout the pregnancy, there is a significant increase in sex steroid hormones such as testosterone and oestrogen (Buckwalter et al., 1999). This study also demonstrates a significant decrease of steroid hormones post pregnancy, even below baseline levels. Therefore, it is clear that as coaches we should take advantage of this period of pregnancy, especially within early stages, to maximize strength levels in an attempt to reduce the detraining effects that occur with time taken off training prior and

after the birth. It could be phrased as a potential overreaching phase. Due to such hormonal changes, there is a fluctuation of mood state throughout, although no statistical correlation has been found between hormonal increase and mood state (Buckwalter et al., 1999). It is important that a coach is aware of the psychological implications during pregnancy and be prepared to alter coaching style. Finally, as the athlete puts on more weight due to the increasing size of the foetus, it should be noted that in sports that load the lower limb joints (e.g. running), greater forces are going to be put through the joints, so caution on volume should be taken.

Measuring menstrual cycle

For optimal results and effective programme design for females, as already mentioned, coaches should know the menstrual cycles of their athletes. Measuring them however, is important and there are ways that could increase the accuracy, which has to be the ultimate aim. Although the average menstrual cycle lasts 28 days and has the phases explained earlier in this chapter, every female athlete is different and a healthy cycle might not consist of the perfect phases and time lengths (Prior and Vignor, 1991). Therefore, there is a need to measure for each athlete individually. Basal body temperature (BBT) patterns can be used to estimate cycles. A 0.2–0.3°C increase in BBT suggests that ovulation has occurred, due to an increase in the levels of progesterone (Vollman, 1977). However, there are limitations with this method (Bauman, 1981), and it is suggested that hormonal levels are the most effective measure (Landgren, Unden, and Diczfalusy, 1980). Within elite and non-elite sport alike, time and cost are an issue and BBT may be the most effective to use if it can be made as accurate as possible (Prior et al., 1990). It is the general rule within elite sport that minimal input should be applied in testing, with

91

maximal output. Therefore, cost and time are not compromised too much although results are extremely useful. Subjective feedback is also a method that can be used from athletes themselves, informing the coach when the athletes enter into certain phases; the coach can then work backwards after that initial date is discovered. The reliability and validity becomes dependent on the athlete and in my opinion, a combination of subjective and objective data is preferable. Once the coach knows the cycle of each athlete, they have the information to plan their training programmes. It is this task that demonstrates how the female population is more complex gender when programming for injury prevention and performance gains. Ensure that you are adaptable, as cycles can fluctuate on a monthly basis and be dependent on many other factors.

SUMMARY

This chapter has explored the differences that occur and problems that can arise for female athletes. First the ways in which common injuries in female athletes can be reduced were discussed. The most common injury documented was to the ACL, and various training modalities can be applied to reduce the risk. Secondly, the Female Athlete Triad was introduced and how energy availability can affect menstrual function and bone strength. Commonly, energy availability is too low in the female population, due to a lack of intake, and good education about optimal intake of energy is essential here. Lastly, the menstrual cycle was covered, and how this can alter training; some essential information was reported on the optimal time to train certain characteristics, and when others need to be reduced. Hormonal fluctuation has a big influence on training intensity and volume. It is clear that coaches need to individualize and programme with a different approach when working with female athletes.

8 | MATURING AND YOUTH ATHLETES

This chapter will assess the various training modalities available for maturing and youth athletes. Prevention of injury at various stages of maturation will be covered, and performance enhancement tools will be outlined. Traditional and more novel theories of maturation and training will be proposed, with a critical analysis of them all, backed up with some personal experience.

Training athletes in the youth age groups is a topic I have been studying and practising for the majority of my coaching career, working predominantly with footballers. My practical experience in providing key coaching techniques complements the theory behind it. This chapter will focus on various aspects of fitness, and demonstrate how using them at particular stages of a maturing athlete's career can reduce injury potential and maximize performance. Myths will also be dispelled about training children, especially when referring to resistance training with maturing athletes.

It is essential that coaches do not treat children like miniature adults: there are clear differences between them (Faigenbaum *et al.*, 2009). This chapter will focus on the development of the original long term athletic development (LTAD) theory, and its evolution over the years. The original theory proposed by Bloom (1985) identified that there were different stages that should be emphasized throughout a child's development. However, the theory was based on an athlete's chronological age. It was later identified and suggested that chronological age wasn't the most accurate method of determining maturing athletes' stages. It was reported that biological age is essential (Balyi and Hamilton, 2004), the biological and physical maturity of an athlete. It is apparent that when working with maturing athletes, regardless of having the same chronological age, their biological ages can be very different, so contrasting approaches need to be taken with each athlete.

Assessing an athlete's biological age takes into account their peak height velocity (PHV). PHV can be calculated fairly accurately and should be a procedure that occurs within sports clubs and organizations to assess each individual in terms of their biological maturation (Balyi and Hamilton, 2004). In boys, PHV occurs on average at 14 years of age in the UK for males, and at 12 years of age for females (Balyi and Hamilton, 2004). It lasts for approximately 2 years and the rate of growth significantly increases, up to 9–11 inches per year (Balyi and Hamilton, 2004). However, this

YOUTH PHYSICAL DEVELOPMENT (YPD) MODEL FOR FEMALES

CHRONOLOGICAL AGE (YEARS)	2	3	4	5	6	7	8	9	10	11	12	13	14	15	16	17	18	19	20	21+
AGE PERIODS	EARLY CHILDHOOD			MIDDLE CHILDHOOD					ADOLESCENCE								ADULTHOOD			
GROWTH RATE	RAPID GROWTH ⟷			STEADY GROWTH ⟷					ADOLESCENT SPURT ⟷					DECLINE IN GROWTH RATE						
MATURATIONAL STATUS					YEARS PRE-PHV ⟵						PHV ⟶				YEARS POST-PHV					
TRAINING ADAPTATION	PREDOMINANTLY NEURAL (AGE-RELATED) ⟷								COMBINATION OF NEURAL AND HORMONAL (MATURITY-RELATED)											
PHYSICAL QUALITIES	FMS			FMS			FMS		FMS											
	SSS			SSS			SSS		SSS											
	Mobility			Mobility					Mobility											
	Agility			Agility					Agility				Agility							
	Speed			Speed					Speed				Speed							
	Power			Power					Power				Power							
	Strength			Strength					Strength				Strength							
	Hypertrophy			Hypertrophy					Hypertrophy		Hypertrophy						Hypertrophy			
	Endurance & MC			Endurance & MC					Endurance & MC				Endurance & MC							
TRAINING STRUCTURE	UNSTRUCTURED			LOW STRUCTURE					MODERATE STRUCTURE				HIGH STRUCTURE				VERY HIGH STRUCTURE			

A visual representation of the YPD Model by Lloyd and Oliver (2012) for females.

YOUTH PHYSICAL DEVELOPMENT (YPD) MODEL FOR MALES

CHRONOLOGICAL AGE (YEARS)	2	3	4	5	6	7	8	9	10	11	12	13	14	15	16	17	18	19	20	21+
AGE PERIODS	EARLY CHILDHOOD			MIDDLE CHILDHOOD						ADOLESCENCE							ADULTHOOD			
GROWTH RATE	RAPID GROWTH ⟷			STEADY GROWTH ⟷						ADOLESCENT SPURT ⟷					DECLINE IN GROWTH RATE					
MATURATIONAL STATUS					YEARS PRE-PHV ⟵							PHV ⟶			YEARS POST-PHV					
TRAINING ADAPTATION	PREDOMINANTLY NEURAL (AGE-RELATED) ⟷									COMBINATION OF NEURAL AND HORMONAL (MATURITY-RELATED)										
PHYSICAL QUALITIES	FMS			FMS				FMS		FMS										
	SSS			SSS				SSS		SSS										
	Mobility			Mobility					Mobility											
	Agility			Agility					Agility				Agility							
	Speed			Speed					Speed				Speed							
	Power			Power					Power				Power							
	Strength			Strength					Strength				Strength							
	Hypertrophy			Hypertrophy					Hypertrophy		Hypertrophy						Hypertrophy			
	Endurance & MC			Endurance & MC						Endurance & MC				Endurance & MC						
TRAINING STRUCTURE	UNSTRUCTURED			LOW STRUCTURE					MODERATE STRUCTURE				HIGH STRUCTURE				VERY HIGH STRUCTURE			

A visual representation of the YPD Model by Lloyd and Oliver (2012) for males.

is just an average and each athlete will go through their PHV at different stages. When athletes go through this PHV phase, they are significantly more likely to get injured, from an overload perspective, and they may have some performance decrement known as 'adolescent awkwardness', which sees a reduction in co-ordination, speed and agility (Philippaerts *et al.*, 2006). Only 25 per cent of maturing athletes, however, suffer from this drop in movement/physical ability.

Ways of calculating PHV have varied over the years, but has more recently been based on an equation looking at the ratio between the standing and seated height of the athlete. It is based on a complex algorithm proposed by Mirwald *et al.* (2002), although a template can be accessed online that requires the height details, in which the PHV measure will be given. Although the underpinning algorithm is too complex for many to understand, please see the equation below (Sherar *et al.*, 2005), which you can use to calculate your athletes' PHV.

Maturity offset = −9.233 + (0.0002708 × leg length and sitting height interaction) + (−0.001663 × age and leg length interaction) + (0.007216 × age and sitting height interaction) + (0.02292 × weight by height ratio)

Obviously to ensure you can use this equation, the variables required from an athlete are: standing height (cm), seated height (cm), date of birth, and weight (kg). It is important that these measures are being taken accurately and consistently for valid and reliable results. It must be appreciated that it is only an estimate and there can be 6 months' variance either side.

When looking at maturity and in reference to tracking growing rates there are other measures that can be done. You can measure the athlete at regular time intervals and track how much they are growing per year within that period. For example, if you measure an athlete's height 4 times year, then you will multiply the difference in height between time points by 4 to gain a cm/year measurement. Then you can visually track the rate of growth and when the curve is at its steepest. However, this approach provides good analysis post growth spurt but cannot predict future rates, so its usefulness within the applied setting is difficult.

Balyi and Hamilton (2004), within their LTAD plan, proposed that there were specific windows of opportunity within a development stage of an athlete, to enhance a specific component of fitness. It was suggested that if the window was missed, then an athlete's maximum potential long term would be hampered in that fitness component. This was however, challenged by strength and conditioning gurus in paediatric development Lloyd and Oliver (2012). Their more recent theory, which is called the youth physical development (YPD) model, suggests that there are not specific windows to optimize particular components of fitness, and that benefits of various components of fitness can be achieved throughout maturation for various reasons. These specific reasons and fitness

components will be discussed in greater detail within this chapter, depicting clear differences between the two theories, and personal opinions based on practical evidence also. Physical qualities discussed below are not in any order of priority.

DEVELOPING STRENGTH

It is now widely accepted that it is safe to perform resistance training within the child population, as long as there is a qualified professional supervising the activity (Baker et al., 2011; Behm et al., 2008; Faigenbaum et al., 2001; Lloyd et al., 2012). Within the LTAD theory (Balyi and Hamilton, 2004), it was suggested that the window of opportunity for increasing strength gains were 12–18 months post PHV. This is related to an athlete's peak weight velocity (PWV) (Beunen and Malina, 2005), and a significantly greater increase in sex steroid hormones such as testosterone, which would elicit greater hypertrophy (Viru et al., 1999). However, Lloyd and Oliver (2012), proponents of the YPD theory, suggest that this theory would limit strength gains to increasing muscle cross-sectional area and developments in muscle mass and hypertrophy. Maximizing strength is multi-faceted and increasing neurological aspects can significantly enhance strength. Therefore, strength training should be prescribed with athletes of low chronological and biological ages as the neural plasticity is higher, and neural development will be enhanced (Borms, 1986). This is reinforced with scientific research that supports the idea that strength can be enhanced with prepubertal and adolescent athletes (Behringer et al., 2010; Behringer et al., 2011). It is important to note that athletes and children will naturally get stronger as they get chronologically and biologically older, and it's hard to attribute the strength gains purely to the training stimulus. However, maximizing strength gains will be a combination of natural growth and training. Maturation alone is not sufficient for impacting performance and injury reduction, and the coach must attempt to get the athlete closer to their genetic ceiling.

As discussed in the first chapter of this book, the importance of maximal strength for performance enhancement and injury prevention is clear. The YPD model in particular demonstrates the importance of strength training at all biological and maturation stages. This is based upon the significant amount of research that suggests higher levels of strength are correlated to higher running speed (Weyand et al., 2000), muscular power (Wisloff et al., 2004), change of direction speed (Negrete and Brophy, 2000), plyometric ability (Miyaguchi and Demura, 2008), and endurance capability (Hoff, Helgerud and Wisloff, 1999). Furthermore, higher levels of strength have been attributed to greater competency level in FMS and its variations (Behringer et al., 2011). It is for this reason that strength training should be an integral part of an athlete's programme. Although not much research has been completed on the maturing athlete, newer research has been published to confirm the importance of strength training. Older research from Teeple et al. (1975) demonstrated that strength accounted for 70 per cent variability for subjects aged 7–12 in various motor skills (jumping, sprinting, throwing). More recent research from Comfort et al. (2014) has identified significant correlations between strength and acceleration/jumping in well trained youth soccer players, even though soccer is not known for its focus on strength training.

Aside from performance variables, the impact on injury potential must not be neglected. Unsurprisingly, high levels of strength have been significantly related to lower injury rates (Faigenbaum et al., 2009). In fact, a combination of high aerobic fitness levels and low strength levels has been suggested optimal for highest injury risk. There is an abundance of academic research that demonstrates the importance of strength training for maturing athletes, at all age groups, both chronologically and biologically. It is therefore astounding that some coaches refrain from introducing young athletes to strength training, even through growth spurt periods, as they believe it will cause injury or they deem it unsafe. It is, in fact, a high volume of endurance and technical/tactical training that aggravates growth related injuries, due to submaximal overload, not strength training within the gym (DiFiori, 1999). However, strength sessions must be programmed and delivered by a qualified professional (UKSCA or equivalent), otherwise the risk of injury could be higher. A detailed LTAD plan for strength development is proposed in Chapter 1, and will be reinforced in a personal long term plan for youth players at the end of this chapter.

Referring back to the original LTAD theory (Balyi and Hamilton, 2004; Bloom, 1985), it was proposed that strength training should be completed post-growth spurt, as a direct indicator of increasing hormonal concentrations such as testosterone (Viru et al., 1999). As we have established, with close reference to the YPD model by Lloyd and Oliver (2012), strength training pre-growth spurt will elicit significant gains due to neurological adaptations. However, if a well-designed strength programme has been delivered to maturing athletes through the system, then post-PHV seems an optimal time to enhance strength via both hypertrophy and neural benefits. Coaches are then urged to utilize this opportunity, building on the strength work performed prior to PHV, and prescribe high intensity and volume strength training to elicit further gains in strength. This higher strength level throughout an athlete's maturation will transfer to the sporting arena, increasing the control of high force/velocity actions.

Although I am an advocate for strength training and the huge benefits it has in reducing injury risk and enhancing performance, it is not always the best modality for every individual. There are many athletes with biomechanical dysfunctions that need to be addressed in the first instance. Applying high load to an individual with dysfunctions could potentially cause further disruption and injury concerns. Therefore, strength training may not be appropriate for these athletes and ensuring they have the correct mobility ranges and stability properties at particular joints should be a priority. A recent article by Bahr (2014) described how maturing athletes can adopt many overuse injuries due to overload within sporting movement patterns, or loading with many dysfunctions. The coach needs to understand that maturing players are still growing and structures aren't fully developed. Of course strength work can have benefits in isolation; however, it needs to be considered within the overall programme and with the individual athlete.

DEVELOPING FUNCTIONAL MOVEMENT SKILLS (FMS)

Fundamental movement skills have been discussed in preceding chapters of this book, specifically when assessing the mobility and stability of an athlete. It has become common practice within elite academies and institutes that FMS are prescribed within early stages of maturation when neural plasticity of the athlete is high. It has been demonstrated that FMS development is essential in teaching correct movement patterns for more specific and complex movements later on (Oliver, Lloyd and Meyers, 2011). They are seen as the building blocks that should develop gross motor skills and a range of physical qualities (Deli, Bakle and Zachopoulou, 2006).

These skills prescribed are primarily performed in the foundation years of development, and should be the main priority of the programme (Lloyd and Oliver, 2012) for athletes aged between 6 and 10. The earlier this type of work is performed, the less corrective exercise techniques a coach will have to do later on. Coaches should focus within this stage on prescribing a broad set of movement patterns, which will challenge the athlete within many physical qualities, such as mobility, stability, posture and so on. The type of coaching and how to deliver these sessions will be discussed later on in this chapter; variation, randomization,

and high levels of interaction should be included within these sessions so there is an unstructured play feel (Lloyd and Oliver, 2012). As athletes mature and progress, it is essential these FMS skills are maintained and consistently performed with older athletes to avoid detraining within these qualities (Lloyd and Oliver, 2012). Optimal times are within warm-ups where high levels of mobility and activation will occur within these movements, also supplementing the warm-up objectives (Jeffreys, 2007). It is important that these movements are as far away from the specific skills of the sport as possible. If we can create athletes who can enhance their movement as a whole, across a wide variety of skills, this will have a significantly greater impact on injury rates and performance. It is important that new challenges are constantly being prescribed, and progression is evident. If the same movements are being prescribed within every session, physical development is limited; it is therefore a coach's priority to be creative and inventive with movement games and sessions.

Mobility

The traditional LTAD model proposes a clear opportunity to develop mobility within maturing athletes of very low chronological age of 5–11 (Malina, 2007), when high priority should be focused on FMS also, as the two often go hand-in-hand. Athletes at this age should already have a high level of suppleness so this should be utilized for maximum results in mobility. The YPD model agrees that 5–11 is the critical age of mobility development (Santos and Janeira, 2008). However, Lloyd and Oliver (2012) propose that at no time should mobility be the main priority of the programme, and that athletes should be focused on being able to achieve the ranges required for their sport. I personally disagree with this, and believe that for some athletes, mobility deficiencies are the cause of increased injury potential, especially within sports that are very repetitive in nature, and require athletes to go through multiple repetitions of short ranges. Here, a natural tightness and lack of movement will be evident at particular joints. Further, in conjunction to development of all other physical qualities, for particular sports and individuals mobility should be a priority of training.

Looking at the work of Kelvin Giles, Michael Boyle and Gray Cook, and the various podcasts and webinars they deliver, the importance of mobility is highlighted. Although these S&C coaches are very successful worldwide, they offer a predominantly corrective exercise/ physiotherapist approach to S&C, which I would be cautious about. Nonetheless, some of their information is very good and I urge readers to explore their work and views, which are easily accessible online. Their view is that ankles, hips and thoracic spine need to be mobile, whilst the knees, lumbar spine and the shoulder need to be stable, in what is known as the joint-by-joint approach. I believe strongly in developing these qualities at particular joints with maturing athletes. As noted before, if there is a lack of mobility or stability within a particular joint it can affect the joint above or below. The most common example in my experience is that a lack of mobility at the ankle can cause a lack of stability at the knee. So injuries occurring at the knee need to be assessed: the cause may not be the knee directly or indeed the surrounding muscle/connective structures – it could be the joint above or below that is the problem. This also provides evidence of how mobility and stability go together, and that high levels of both are essential for the optimal moving athlete. As mentioned before, there are some exceptions in particular sports. For example, long distance runners require extremely stiff ankles for efficient transfer of elastic energy through the Achilles tendon. If athletes are pain-free, mobility may not be a quality targeted as performance would be negatively impacted, although this would need to be assessed on an individual basis.

Physical literacy

Kelvin Giles (mentioned briefly above), adopts a unique approach that contradicts traditional S&C ideologies: he suggests that getting athletes stronger and adding more load is not necessarily the best way to produce healthy robust athletes who don't break down. Instead, his approach focuses on enhancing the quality of movement and challenging the athletes differently in a physical way. Firstly, it is important that an athlete can perform basic movement patterns such as the ability to squat on two legs and on one (it is astounding to see athletes who can squat twice their bodyweight bilaterally, but cannot control the simplest task unilaterally). Other movement patterns such as lunging, bracing, pushing, and pulling are proposed. These foundation exercises should then be prescribed in all directions and all planes. Giles criticizes Olympic weightlifting techniques as they lack the ability to be performed in multiple planes and directions. I would counteract this argument, however, as Olympic lifting is prescribed to enhance physiological ability to express force quickly, in a triple extension pattern. (My opinions are reinforced in a programme template for the maturing athlete at the end of this chapter.)

Much of Giles's research has been carried out in the U.S. by interspersing small pockets of physical literacy movement work throughout a P.E. or classroom session. This has proved effective in the acquisition of motor patterns, as the sessions are randomized and varied – two key variables that are essential for the development of physical literacy within maturing athletes. Another concept proposed for maturing athletes is the need for game-based learning. In contrast to very structured drills that teach the athletes a particular movement pattern in an external way with cued coaching, game-based learning requires problem solving and intrinsic learning to provide the best solution. This has been proposed optimal for long term skill and cognitive development. I believe a combination of both is essential throughout: cues and corrective exercise techniques are at times important, but the coach has to provide the opportunity for the athlete to solve the puzzle initially.

Originally, physical literacy ideas were adopted in Canada by Higgs *et al.* (2008), who proposed that physical literacy was the ability of an athlete to develop fundamental movement and sport skills that an athlete can perform confidently and under control. It also included the ability to read and react to certain situations effectively. This highlights the importance of cognitive function, reinforcing Giles's theory about physical literacy within S&C. It is often neglected when prescribing and delivering S&C sessions to athletes, that athletes will have to react to a stimulus within sport and perform a particular movement pattern. If this cognitive function is missed out, then the transfer of movement work to the competitive environment will be limited, so movement enhancement and injury prevention will be reduced. This is reinforced in the theory of non-linear pedagogy and the constraints theory, which develop important ideas about how skills are learnt and effectively transferred into sporting and competitive environments. The reader is referred to Chow *et al.*, (2008) and Newell (1986) for further information regarding this approach.

Metabolic conditioning

Original LTAD models have suggested maturing athletes either side of PHV can achieve significant gains in metabolic conditioning, assessed by aerobic endurance and VO2 max scores (Baquet, Van Praagh and Berthoin, 2003). The YPD model, however (Lloyd and Oliver, 2012), suggests a controversial approach, that at no stage during maturation should an athlete's programme be focused on endurance capacities. It is the case with the majority of children that they will perform extremely high volumes of submaximal locomotion within specific sport technical/tactical training and within daily function. Physical education teachers will often include a form of submaximal aerobic work within their lessons, as it is deemed

safer than high intensity resistance training. In fact, the majority of non-impact injuries within children and adolescents are due to significant overload of submaximal exercise (DiFiori, 1999). Injuries specifically to tendons or other connective structures occur when overloaded through a high volume of training and an immature development of connective structures. This reinforces the importance of reducing any endurance-based exercise at the maturing athlete level, until full development of the body has occurred. However, some energy system development is important within maturation as physiological fitness can otherwise be limited in the long term.

PUTTING THEORIES AND OPINIONS INTO A LONG-TERM PLAN

Having reviewed much research and explored the most popular and creditable athlete plans for the maturing athlete, I have outlined a new plan below, based on a combination of a number of experts' proposals. As often discussed, the main focus will be geared towards injury prevention, although performance will often be improved as a by-product when increasing certain physical qualities.

Phase 1 (Foundation): 7–11

Within this initial phase, the practitioner has a number of years with which to build the foundations for athletic potential later on. These years, therefore, are essential for an athlete's ability to withstand injuries effectively. The first foundation phase will in particular be similar to a physical literacy approach, and the theories proposed by Kelvin Giles. Therefore, it is suggested that a broad set of movement skills are prescribed to athletes of this age, including a high volume of FMS and their variations, as well as various locomotor skills. It is essential that skills and exercises are prescribed in every direction and every plane for a fully developed acquisition of a particular skill. It is also essential that various skills are performed with huge variation and randomization, although working to various planned frameworks behind the scenes.

All qualities should be developed through dynamic exercises in challenging positions, so the need for specific mobility work is not necessary at this stage. If possible, all movement work should be completed in small blocks throughout a technical session if possible. Interspersing small pockets of movement work creates greater skill acquisition and motor patterns long term as the athletes have to retrieve the relevant schema in a randomized order. All or nearly all of sessions should be prescribed within a game-based approach, whether this be a type of race, or creative game that looks to enhance a particular quality. Favour implicit learning and problem solving over extrinsic coaching cues, and endorse analogies that provide an effective response and interaction from the young athlete. Try to encourage the athlete to come up with optimal solutions of the correct way of moving before giving any specific cues to improve. This is not to say, however, that coaches should not coach; if an athlete needs to improve technique in an area, then they should be cued. Can you be clever in your coaching to drive the correct solution without telling them directly? Sessions should portray a 'play' like nature, and appear largely unstructured. Although sessions look like they are disorganised and chaotic, do not let this confuse or mislead you. Lots of chaos is a good sign for skill acquisition at this stage, although ensuring they are competent in various movement skills is important.

At the end of Phase 1 an athlete should have a good physical literacy, with the ability to perform a variety of movement tasks in a multitude of directions and planes. They should have developed basic gross motor skills (running, shuffling, catching, throwing, co-

ordination, etc.) and developed good single leg stability. Various cognitive skills should have been developed through a host of decision-making tasks within various games. This cognitive aspect of performance is essential, and should be prescribed prior to any structured technical work.

Phase 2 (Physical development phase): 12–14

Once athletes have passed the foundation phase, the next phase can provide a more structured programme on the various physical qualities to be enhanced. This stage is essential as it is when the majority of male athletes are going through their growth spurt, i.e. between −1 and 1 on the APHV scale. This stage will be split into three different areas: the locomotor emphasis on the pitch/court/sporting arena; prehab modalities; and gym-based competencies.

Locomotor qualities

After the previous phase, athletes should have a good foundation of locomotor skills, in all planes and directions. This next phase looks to enhance all these qualities in greater detail. The first quality that should be emphasized initially, which underpins the technical and physical performance of other locomotor skills, is deceleration and landing mechanics. These are termed eccentric control locomotor skills, and will enhance the ability to control eccentric load efficiently. Then specific work can be done on acceleration and top speed mechanics, change of direction and variations of sideways/backwards movements. In this age group, movements should be fairly generic, not sports-specific.

The aim of this phase is to ensure that technical aspects of various movements are enhanced. Therefore, greater detail should be evident in coaching sessions, aiming to improve the control of and efficiency of movement (it is called 'neuromuscular training'). There should be greater structure at times but variation should be applied; a combination of more structure with some chaotic drills is required for achieving effective transfer to the sporting environment. Challenge the athlete initially with a closed skill, then an open one, through to chaos to develop cognitive function, closely associated with greater control in agility and plyometric elements. Challenging PHV athletes with high cognitive elements is essential.

For those athletes who struggle when going through their main growth spurt, complexity of tasks may be reduced and it may be necessary to re-programme and revisit some basic motor patterning with the athletes' new limb lengths. Prescribing highly challenging cognitive drills before the growth spurt can limit the detrimental effect it has on things like co-ordination. Ensure an athlete is also mobile and stable going into a growth spurt; this will also provide a better foundation for the body coping with rapid change.

Prehab modalities

Having worked with physiotherapists, and within a multi-disciplinary team, my knowledge of prehab modalities has significantly increased. It is essential at this age group, if we want to start adding load in the following years, that athletes are made more stable and more mobile. I used to believe we should make athletes more mobile first, then adding stability and strength. It now comes apparent that a lack of stability can limit an athlete's active mobility. For example, an athlete may have high passive mobility in hip flexion lying on a bench; however, when they are asked to perform hip flexion tasks on one leg, such as a single leg squat, their mobility is impaired because they are not stable enough to reach full hip flexion capabilities. Therefore, mobility and stability should be developed simultaneously.

Modalities for enhancing mobility include a thorough stretching programme, with various static and dynamic movements. Three key areas are the ankle, hip, and thoracic spine. Although research is mixed or very limited, foam rolling is provided in programmes for my athletes, to reduce acute tightness and any exercise-induced stress within the muscles, and to increase range at particular joints. It is often used to increase the perception of freshness within the athletes, so may be a psychological enhancement as opposed to physiological. Key FMS exercises are still essential for developing mobility in a dynamic way, and are more engaging and interactive for athletes if delivered well.

Increasing stability is where the S&C coach and physiotherapist collide; however, I have tried to compromise and incorporate a combined effective stability programme. It is essential that athletes have a high volume and variation of glute exercises to enhance hip stability, and that these muscles can be switched on within movements, otherwise the hip flexors/hamstrings will take too much load and be at greater risk of injury, or cause lower back pain. Various exercises such as glute bridges, clamshells, and laying abduction are good examples of glute exercises. (A list of specific glute exercises was provided in Chapter 1, along with different variations to activate the three muscles within the glutes.) The coach is urged to ensure these muscles are being activated and the athlete isn't compensating with other global stabilizers. It is important that athletes can tolerate a high volume of these exercises as this will be the best way to adapt. Secondly, it is important to integrate that glute activation after an isolated exercise in a squatting or other dynamic pattern, bilaterally initially, then unilaterally. This is where the link to the gym-based competencies occurs.

Single leg stability is essential, ensuring an athlete can balance effectively on one leg initially, moving onto some single leg squatting patterns and eccentric control. This provides good control of the knee and ankle when combined with the landing work performed in the locomotor sessions. The last aspect within stability is the control of the trunk. Initially within this stage the athlete should become familiar with the dissociation of the pelvis, completing pelvic tilts. Encourage full flexion/extension in a quadrupedal position so activation of the key trunk muscles occur. This also gets the athletes used to the neutral position at the stage in-between the movements of the tilts. Also, provide exercises such as superman drills, which encourage activation of the trunk as a whole to stabilize movements of the arm/leg. Ensure that the athlete can now hold neutral spinal position throughout the exercise. This creates the foundations for developing high levels of stiffness in the next phase.

Gym-based competencies

Although at the foundation stage many gym-based movements were incorporated within the field-based physical literacy sessions, this will be the first time athletes will be introduced to the gym. For me, the development of strength begins with being competent in various movement patterns within the gym. All of these technical movements should be performed with no load originally and there is no rush over the next three years to apply load. Obviously, if athletes become very competent at certain movements, do not be afraid to add load. This is where individualized programmes become essential.

The key patterns that are essential to learn are: squatting (overhead, front, back), deadlifts, hinging techniques focusing on hamstring conditioning such as RDLs and Nordic curls, a multi-directional lunge, combined with other single leg stability exercises. For the upper body, pushes and pulls in both vertical/horizontal planes are recommended. These competencies, practised over three years, should provide an extremely effective base for strength development, along with the effective prehab modalities performed.

This is a key phase in the athlete's growth, and as growth-related injuries could potentially be a lot higher, metabolic conditioning should be significantly reduced. There should be no emphasis on increasing endurance capacities within any S&C focus, and technical/tactical coaches should be aware of the load an athlete is going through when they are between −1 and +1 in their APHV. Attention within this period also needs to be drawn towards tendons and other connective structures that may not be fully developed. Coaches may reduce the amount of high intensity locomotor work (such as bounding/deceleration etc.) within this period to avoid the onset of any overload issues. A re-visit of various motor skills may be required if an athlete suffers what is known as adolescent awkwardness when going through their growth spurt. Assessing this, however, is very subjective so the coach needs to put on his art cap and watch the movement of his players. High volumes of training should be avoided at this stage.

Phase 3 (Sports-specific physical development): 15–16

If the athlete and coach have been fortunate enough to follow a long-term plan for eight years they can now be progressed physically.

Locomotor skills

Within the sport arena, the athlete should have developed a good technical model for many different movements, especially within a closed skill scenario. Within this next phase, it is essential that these skills are incorporated within more sports-specific drills. However, closed drills should be still present in the programme and the key movements that would be essential for reducing injuries have to be reinforced, i.e. decelerating, landing mechanics and change of direction. All other locomotor skills are aimed more at an improvement in performance. Try to increase the stress of these important skills for further adaptation if the athlete is technically competent.

Prehab modalities

With all athletes potentially having good mobility and stability it is essential that programmes are now individualized. Being realistic, we know some athletes will still not have the best mobility and stability, due to the constant high volume of sporting actions with short ROM being performed. The groups I would suggest for individualized prehab modalities would then be mobility (ankle, hip, and T-spine) and stability (ankle, knee, shoulder and trunk). The trunk work can now progress to exercises such as planks where the aim is to increase stiffness of the trunk for longer durations. This can be done with all players within prehab sessions. Therefore, players could be in a sub-group from every category working on that particular area. This will look to be more specific with these age groups within prehab modalities, based on either subjective or objective measures.

Gym-based competencies

After becoming competent in the various gym-based movements in the previous phase, exercises should now be progressed to generate a greater physiological/neurological adaptation. Getting athletes stronger in squatting, single leg, hamstring conditioning, upper body push and pulls will now have a great effect within their sport. As well as these higher force exercises, it is essential that the high velocity exercises are progressed, challenging athletes now in higher box jumps, both single and double limb, increasing their reactive strength through depth jumps and adding a multidirectional ability also. Regardless of biological age, athletes should be loaded up in this phase, if advanced and competent enough to do so. However, the coach must be aware of late developers who are still going through PHV, and have growth issues. Many athletes at this chronological or biological age, 18 months post-PHV, may well take advantage of a greater

hormonal increase, so greater hypertrophy could be a possibility if desired within the athlete. If an athlete is pre-PHV then neurological gains will still provide increase in strength.

Phase 4 (maximizing genetic potential): 17+

This phase should be the easiest one, if the preceding phases have been done effectively. After the chronological age of 17, the majority of athletes should have gone through their main PHV. Therefore, this is now the right opportunity to maximize all physical qualities within strength and conditioning programmes. Ensure that programmes are regressed with the minority of athletes who are still in their PHV phase.

Within the gym it is essential, now athletes have good motor patterns and are mobile and stable, that they are progressed and overloaded with strength and power training. Strength and power significantly reduce injury rates, so must be prioritized in programmes. The categories were important to provide the athlete with the tools and foundations to now begin more advanced S&C programmes.

Within locomotor skills, maximum performance should be a priority as well as still enhancing movement quality and technique for greater efficiency within the sporting arena. It is interesting now, that all other movements will still be enhanced as previously discussed, although metabolic conditioning can be prescribed in significantly higher volumes. Whereas it has been proposed inappropriate and unnecessary to prescribe metabolic conditioning to athletes younger than this age, now is the time to develop high levels of anaerobic/aerobic endurance, not only because of increasing performance but if an athlete has a higher level of endurance, they can handle more training volume in general, making them less likely to break down within certain phases. Obviously the sport itself will dictate whether high levels of endurance are necessary, but if you feel it is, now is the time to design and enhance these qualities through your programme. However, no matter what sport you are in, if you require aerobic endurance, the athlete must be hit with both a central and peripheral adaptation. If one only is hit, then this will limit the endurance capabilities of the athlete and pose a greater risk to injury.

Prehab modalities should stay individualized, and should depend on what that athlete needs, based on the consequences of performing repetitive patterns within their sport. In the majority of sports certain prehab modalities will always have to be performed. For example, mobility work, glute activation and trunk training will be modalities that are always required. However, it is up to the S&C coach to effectively progress these qualities and drive further adaptation for the athlete to become structurally stronger.

This phase, similar to the one proposed by Lloyd and Oliver (2012) should be a lot more structured, especially within the S&C aspects. It was mentioned that with earlier phases, sessions should be cognitively challenging and have a varied and randomized approach. However, I feel athletes should get specific cognitive development through sports-specific skills within technical and tactical training. Therefore, key communication is required with the technical/tactical coach to develop drills and sessions that incorporate high cognitive elements. Other S&C elements can be more structured, and greater emphasis on increasing a particular physical quality should be applied.

TRAINING AGE

The proposed long term development plan above, based on theory and experience working with these age groups, can only be applied fully if a coach has the athlete from very young, and all the way through the system. Clearly this isn't always the case, and when athletes come into your system at various ages, training age becomes more important than

biological or chronological age. Nonetheless, biological age is important and will dictate particular training modalities. There is a need for the school curriculum to provide the foundations of movement and physical literacy so all athletes and children are exposed to essential motor patterns and skills at young ages.

INDIVIDUALIZATION

The most important aspect of working with any athlete, but particularly younger athletes, is providing a high level of individualization within programmes, based on their biological age and capability. This obviously depends on resources and personnel with younger age groups, or even older athletes at particular clubs and institutes. The coach therefore needs to be creative to develop the individual and their needs and remember that one size doesn't fit all.

This chapter acknowledges Bloom (1985), and Balyi and Hamilton (2004), for original theories on long term athlete development, and Lloyd and Oliver (2012) for their ongoing research and proposal of the youth physical development model that has had a huge influence on my own long term plans. The plan outlined here provides an effective tool for injury prevention, and describes how certain qualities will underpin reduction in injuries at different stages of development. Biological age is a key area that needs further research, to understand in greater detail the effects that could potentially occur within training environments. One key point I would like to enforce is that with young athletes, unlike adults, a more cautious approach needs to be taken. We should consider not just the physiological stress, but other sociological and psychological components that maturing athletes face through the years. Therefore, a need to undercook training as a whole would be an optimal approach and philosophy when working with children. The minimal dose response is a theory and philosophy I heavily endorse.

9 | THE PHYSIOLOGY MODULE

The title of this chapter is somewhat tongue in cheek as there are obviously elements of both physiology and biomechanics running through all aspects of strength and conditioning. For example, periodization and cycling of physiological load, as well as muscle contraction and force production are physiological aspects of S&C. This chapter, however, will look in more detail at the issues that our athletes face physiologically when competing, which as S&C coaches we need to consider in order to provide appropriate training or prepare our athletes for optimal performance, limiting the incidence of injury. Topics that will be discussed within this chapter are: the importance of sleep and circadian rhythms, the effect of travel, and training/competing in extreme conditions such as the heat and the cold. These more physiological topics are discussed to assist coaches in preparing athletes, keeping them as 'fresh' as possible for performance. The last part of this chapter will then divert away from physiological topics and will assess some practical strategies regarding immunology within sport, and minimizing illness amongst athletes.

THE IMPORTANCE OF SLEEP

The importance of sleep within elite sport, for both enhanced performance and recovery, is now well established within sports science teams (Reilly, 2006). Before the issue of sleep is discussed further, it is important to discuss the body's natural circadian rhythm, which can drive the sleep–wake cycle. The circadian rhythm shows fluctuations in the athlete's performance levels throughout the day, mainly attributed to the natural fluctuation of body temperature (Atkinson and Reilly, 1996). It is proposed that complex motor skills tend to peak earlier in the day, whereas gross motor skills peak at later points, due to an earlier acrophase in alertness as opposed to body temperature increase (Reilly et al., 2005). This immediately challenges the strength and conditioning coach as there are now two optimal parts of the day to gain maximal adaptations. Firstly, it is apparent that higher levels of testosterone occur in the morning, and greater adaptation can be made in strength/hypertrophy by utilizing this increase in sex steroid hormone (Resko and Eik-Nes, 1966). However, based on the circadian rhythm, strength demonstrates an increase at both 13:00 and 16:00 hours within the day due to peaks in body temperature (Reilly and Edwards, 2006), providing a rationale for prescribing strength sessions in the afternoon. Obviously, the schedule of strength and conditioning will most likely work around the technical/tactical programme, but the research above provides food for thought. The circadian rhythm model is based on the athlete waking up at 7:00 hours on average, and having 8 hours of sleep the night before, so adjustment and consideration needs to be made in other circumstances. This rhythm is based on the sleep–wake cycle, predominately on the light and dark hours, and disruption of this normal cycle, such as through lack of sleep or shift patterns causes differences within the cycle.

There are many studies that show the effects of deprived sleep on performance. Thomas and Reilly (1975) demonstrated that it was possible to match 100 hours of non-stop cycling intensity. Energy intake was provided to specifically match the expenditure, delivered in a glucose syrup drink. However, despite the power output being matched, there was a significant reduction in heart rate over 48 hours, which meant that a reduction of sympathetic drive occurred, as well as decreases in lung function tests (forced vital capacity and forced expiratory volume). Furthermore, there were significant reductions in visual reaction time after the first night's sleep loss, and the short-term memory was affected after the second night without sleep. These findings were supported within the research paradigm (Reilly and George, 1983), in that cognitive parameters are most affected by acute sleep loss. Variables such as strength seem to be unaffected after a day's sleep loss, so provides sports that are strength dominant with some flexibility within your athletes' sleep patterns. However, optimal practice would recognize the importance of sleep to recovery, and those athletes who require heavy resistance training would elicit maximal adaptations if their sleep patterns were good (Reilly and Edwards, 2006).

In sports that require potential chronic sleep loss, like ultra-endurance events or sailing events, this is an issue that cannot be avoided. Obviously, these long durations would cause significant reductions in physical and mental performance (Smith and Reilly, 2005). Stampi et al. (1990), proposed the optimal solution for prolonged periods of sleep deprivation. His strategy was implemented with multiple medal winning Ellen MacArthur, who split her sleep into short naps of 25–40 minutes. After all chores and checks were completed, and as long as the weather was satisfactory she would return to sleep for another nap. This technique was hailed as a breakthrough as her physical and cognitive performance were enhanced. Having a power nap for approximately 20 minutes has been demonstrated extremely effective for increasing performance and alertness levels (Hayashi et al., 1999), and should be utilized not only when sleep restriction occurs within an athlete, but on a regular basis if possible. The cultural protocols of many Mediterranean and European countries seem to have an optimal routine with the siesta mid-afternoon, breaking up the working day.

Research on sleep has been predominately on the impact of performance, and there have been very few studies to assess the effects on injury rates. There may be a couple of reasons for this: firstly, sleep studies are very hard to administer as there are so many variables that need controlling in order for it to be valid. Within sporting environments it is extremely hard to ensure all variables are controlled and that the injury rates are due to the lack of sleep, not something else. Secondly, many of those clubs or organizations carrying out studies don't want to release information and prefer to keep the data for internal use. Based on my own experience, there seems to be a correlation between lack of sleep and either illness or injury. Although measuring of sleep has always been subjective, and the injury rate or illness could have occurred from many other sources, there seems to be a trend that three consecutive poor nights' sleep (less than 8 hours) can promote an increased risk of injury or illness. This is not published research however, just an observation from my experience.

Listed below are factors that can further influence athlete performance following sleep loss (Smith and Reilly, 2005):

- Extreme circadian rhythms (morning/ evening types)
- Decreased motivation
- Decreased physical:cognitive task ratio
- Increased duration of task
- Increased complexity of task
- Lower body temperature

Based on these factors I would suggest the following: decrease training duration, provide training in regular times of the day, ensure body temperature is elevated, and decrease the cognitive complexity of the task. It is essential that the sports scientist or S&C coach relays this to the technical/tactical coach if a lack of sleep is evident within your athlete. Another suggestion would be getting them to have a nap (as suggested earlier), and make use of pharmacological compounds such as caffeine which is used as a stimulant.

In an ideal scenario, sleep would be monitored effectively and it would be ensured that athletes are in a regular cycle or rhythm of good sleep. However, we know that this isn't always possible as the control over athletes is not sufficient to monitor them full-time, and they need to take responsibility for their own habits at times. Therefore, if sleep deprivation occurs the S&C coach/sports scientist must act accordingly to prevent it causing any disruption to training and increasing injury/illness risk. Another example of where the circadian rhythm is disrupted is when travelling across multiple time zones, which will be the next section within this chapter.

THE STRESS OF TRAVEL

Over the last fifty years or so, with sport going globalized, and technology advancing, athletes have had the opportunity to travel for sporting competition and/or training camps within their sport. With this travel, athletes and support staff have a high level of excitement, going away from their normal place of work, but may also experience high levels of stress and there may be physiological consequences associated with health and function. The immediate stress of the preparation and flight itself is known as travel fatigue, and it is associated with many variables that will be discussed in this chapter. Travelling across multiple time zones causes not only travel fatigue, but jet lag also, which will also be discussed in greater detail. Many sports scientists do not understand the difference between the two, and how to optimize recovery from bouts of travelling. This section on the stress of travel will provide some support for overcoming both travel fatigue and jet lag, and is based on research findings of Waterhouse, Reilly, and Edwards (2004).

Travel fatigue

Travel fatigue essentially means 'travel weariness' and the effects an individual could suffer when travelling (using any mode of transport) for a period of time. Many symptoms associated with travel fatigue are: general fatigue, disorientation, and headaches. These are caused by disrupting the normal routine, hassles around checking in and baggage claim, and dehydration due to dry cabin air within planes (Waterhouse *et al.*, 2002). Advice on how to overcome these issues will be explained below. Many of these points may not be scientific or academic; however, they are important when working with athletes in an applied setting.

Training recommendations to travel fatigue

Even with flights as short as two hours and not crossing any time zone, the practitioner needs to understand the effects travelling can have. If an athlete has taken a flight that day, then any physical exertion or training should be avoided for that day, and potentially another, so a full day of rest occurs before the athlete resumes their normal training routine. If an athlete is governed to play/compete by a prescribed schedule out of the hands of the support staff, then serious modifications should be taken in the days after to promote recovery and regeneration and ensure the athlete is as close to their normal homeostasis levels as possible. Other implications that need to be considered are the time of the flight, the stress and preparation leading up to it and so on.

Before the flight

It is firstly essential that any preparations are completed thoroughly, and on time; it is also preferable for administration staff to take care of some of the arrangements – things such as ensuring the passport is valid, all health checks are completed, suitable clothing is packed, and so on. It is my opinion that the manager(s) of the athlete or group of athletes should take responsibility for ensuring this all happens efficiently, to reduce the level of stress on the day. The flight organization itself is important: for example, make sure the flight time is optimal, and that any stop-overs are limited (Tsai *et al.*, 1988). Early booking of flights might also allow better seating with greater leg room. The organization on the day must ensure that everyone arrives with plenty of time so no last-minute rushing around has to occur. It is suggested that being properly prepared for travel significantly reduces anxiety levels of athletes (Bor, 2003).

During the flight

The flight cabin itself, particularly in economy class, provides very limited space for passengers. It has been demonstrated that the immobility can cause a lack of circulation and even cramps within athletes. This is known as 'economy class syndrome' (Brown *et al.*, 2001) and can be avoided by regular movement around the cabin and stretching of lower limb muscles throughout. It is also apparent that the air is pressurized and very dry and can cause dehydration, dry lips and a sore mouth. Athletes should therefore take on plenty of fluids, and avoid alcohol and caffeine, which can cause further loss of fluids due to their diuretic properties. Boredom has to also be taken into account, and keeping athletes entertained can be challenging. Sleeping/napping can pass the time, but only if it is a night flight. If it is not then you should strongly advise athletes not to sleep for over an hour, as further disruption to the circadian rhythm and body clock will occur when arriving at the new destination.

After the flight

On arrival at the destination, baggage needs to be claimed, passport checks have to be made, and onward travel to the destination has to occur. This all takes further time and can aggravate the athletes further. Patience and plenty of fluids and reassurance are needed to keep the athletes calm. Many also require a sleep after travel, which again is fine if it is night time, but if you arrive during the day, it is recommended that a nap of no longer than one hour is taken; a shower can help alertness and mood without hindering the sleep of that night (De Looy *et al.*, 1988).

Jet lag

When travelling with athletes across several time zones, as well as the travel fatigue affecting athletes, jet lag also poses a problem. The jet lag phenomenon occurs due to a lack of synchronization of the body clock; adjustment to the new time zone needs to be made. Effective synchronization is completed by the use of 'Zeitgebers', a German term meaning 'time-givers'. This is achieved by potentially manipulating the environment, and altering the light–dark cycle so a gradual synchronization occurs (Waterhouse, 2001). Trying to achieve adjustment instantaneously can actually have a negative impact for longer. The effects of jet lag can be seen within individuals and can develop strange sensations when undertaking normal activities. Symptoms include general tiredness and wakefulness at night, lower concentration, decreased mental and physical performance, increased irritability, and loss of appetite (Waterhouse et al., 1997). Unfortunately, the majority of the symptoms are unavoidable but there are ways to increase the recovery from it. The use of bright light, or inhibiting it through use of sunglasses, can be an effective way to manipulate the environment and adjust from the old light–dark cycle to the new one. Taking small naps when feeling extremely tired (less than 30 minutes) is preferable to sleeping for prolonged periods of time and delaying the synchronization. It is suggested that the new time is set on the athlete's watch before travelling as this will help to mentally deal with such a big change. There is also some theory around using melatonin supplements, as it is generally secreted naturally within the body when the human is in their night mode, between 21:00 and 7:00. Melatonin is said to make adjustments easier when travelling east and night time might be delayed; research, however, demonstrates very mixed views and there is no conclusive evidence to support its effectiveness.

It is essential to know that the approximate effect of jet lag lasts one day for every time zone you cross, as a general rule. This provides the coach and sports science staff with enough information to make sure there is enough time to travel and overcome jet lag prior to competition. It also suggests that if training camps are being organized, going too far away for short durations will not be the best solution and will reduce the quality of training on arrival and return to home. It is worth noting that travelling eastwards takes longer to adjust and this should be taken into account.

Training recommendations to jet lag

Travelling for longer durations and across time zones obviously impact on athletes returning to training schedule. There have to be modifications when the athlete reaches a new destination or returns to the normal training environment. If an athlete has gone through a medium to long duration flight (>4 hours), it is essential that at least two days are allowed for recovery, and the aim would be the get the athlete as close to the new sleep cycle prior to training. After approximately two days full rest, the athlete is integrated into two days modified training, with lower volumes and intensities of work within the training schedule. Following this, it is down to the assessment of the sports science and medical staff to determine whether the athlete is ready to return to full training. Remember, each case is taken on an individual basis, and this is when the art and experience of this job comes into it. If the athlete responds poorly to travel, then it is important that more caution is taken, and the player's wellbeing is looked after prior them to resuming full training.

THE STRESS OF HEAT

There are many sporting events across the globe that take place in extreme heat, which can have an adverse effect on physiological performance. The effect of heat, or change in climate, is often underestimated and there have been a huge number of sporting activities in the past where athletes were affected by this. This section will look at the effects that heat can have on an athlete physiologically, as well as strategies to prepare the athlete for competition in the heat.

It is widely apparent that mainly endurance exercise is impaired in the heat. There seems to be a significant correlation between performance decrement and heat increase (Galloway and Maughan, 1997). The optimum temperature within the laboratory seems to be around 10°C (Maughan and Shireffs, 2004), so this raises the question whether any temperature above this will have a negative impact on performance. It then comes down to the athlete who is most prepared in the environment conditions, as opposed to their physiological profile.

The reduction in performance in the heat is in part due to progressive dehydration that results from sweat loss; remember that sweat loss is body's way of cooling down, although will lead to impaired cardiovascular and thermoregulatory function (Gonzales-Alonso et al., 1999). Ways to overcome and monitor dehydration will be discussed in greater detail later on in this chapter. It is also proposed that reduced performance could be down to an impaired central nervous system (CNS) and not localized at muscular level (Nielsen et al., 2001). Davis et al. (2000) demonstrated that pharmaceutical interventions can limit CNS fatigue in the heat. Gonzales-Alonso et al. (1999b) have proposed that although the environment stress of heat has a further impact on impaired performance, it is actually the core temperature of the athlete reaching a critical 34°C that has been shown to cause a reduction in performance. Therefore, the heat will cause the critical core temperature to be reached earlier.

Acclimation vs. acclimatization

When preparing for competing in the heat, there are two different methods that are utilized to optimize preparation for athletes. It is known that repeated exposure to the heat results in physiological adaptations, which reduce the impact of environment stress on performance (Nielsen et al., 1993). As briefly mentioned above, the two factors that determine the effectiveness of adaptation are the rise in body and core temperature, and the sweating response (Maughan and Shirreffs, 2004). Adaptation depends on the volume and intensity prescribed within the period, which would primarily depend on the sport, event, and individual. However, regardless of whether acclimation or acclimatization occurs, the period it takes for effective adaptation is 14 days, so living and training in hot climates for prolonged periods won't be beneficial; in fact due to a decrease in intensity it may be detrimental to performance.

Acclimatization refers to when the athlete is actually taken to the destination of the event or an equivalent hot climate to adapt. A possible limitation of travelling to a destination where the heat is so high constantly is that the intensity of the sessions for a prolonged duration could be compromised. This is due to the consequences the stress of heat has on exercise performance. Consequently, detraining could occur in an athlete relying solely on acclimatization. One solution might be to find an air-conditioned training facility with a high speed treadmill, where some intensity sessions can be performed in addition to the ones in the heat outside. As mentioned previously, the programme of volume and intensity is entirely down to the type of athlete, sport, event and so on. The consequences of travel fatigue and/or jet lag must be taken into account: training volume and intensity must be reduced in the first few days of arrival at least, to minimize injury, fatigue, etc. The body clock also has to adjust to the new time zone effectively to increase performance and minimize injury. When competing in a hot climate it would be necessary for an athlete to become acclimatized to the new environment; however, there is another method that can have additional benefits when adjusting to performing in the heat.

Acclimation is when an athlete adjusts to the heat in their own environment, but performs additional training within a laboratory, where they add heat training sessions in. It is recommended that an additional heat training session is performed second, and should be more of a volume session as opposed to the high intensity quality work that is done earlier in the day. One session every three days has been proposed as sufficient, for a two-week period. Problems around this method include the fact that it depends on the facilities on offer to the athlete, and a heat laboratory is required. The conditions also need to be matched according to the weather conditions of the destination – a minimum of 30°C but no more than 35°C is recommended – as well as matching the humidity of the lab. Both methods have been proposed and it is in fact a combination of the two that would be optimal for athlete preparation. Leading into the competition five

weeks out, it would be recommended that two weeks incorporated some acclimation, where extra sessions in the lab are performed every three days (minimum). Three weeks leading into the competition the athlete should fly to the venue or one close by to go through their acclimatization phase, prior to completion. Due to an acclimation phase having already being completed, the effects in the new environment should be lessened, and should therefore reduce the modifications to the training schedule in the final phase, although jet lag and other factors need consideration. The work of Maughan and Shirreffs (2004) is acknowledged in the discussion above.

HYDRATION

As discussed earlier in the book (Chapter 2), and touched on within the heat section above, the effects of hydration on exercise performance, fatigue, injury and illness have been reported. This is further heightened with the chance of heat illness in such hot environments. A common misconception is that due to the athletes acclimatizing to the heat, less fluid is required, but the opposite is the case. An important adaptation process to the heat is an increased sweating response; therefore more fluid is required (Sawka and Pandolf, 1990). Although drinks that contain glycogen and electrolytes that were lost within the exercise bout are preferred (Shirreffs *et al.*, 1996), it is important that the rehydration strategies are individualized as some might need more than others. This reduces the chance of athletes putting on unnecessary weight. Aside from monitoring the osmolality of the urine, pre- and post-exercise weighing can be done, to assess how much fluid the body has lost. Although this method has flaws, in my experience it has been effective in reducing dehydration heat illness.

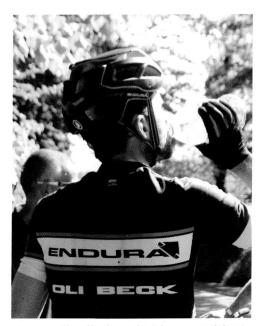

For every 1kg of bodyweight, it is suggested that 1 litre of fluid needs to be replaced.

EXERCISE IN THE COLD

Whereas the last section discussed the issues associated with performing in the heat, consideration must be given to extremes of cold. Defining what cold actually is, however, seems to be a difficult task, although the optimal temperature for performance seems to be around 10–11°C, identified with performance tests in the laboratory (Nimmo, 2004). Temperatures above and below this temperature then demonstrate a linear decrease in performance. It must be noted for those working or aspiring to work within particular sports, that the human body loses heat 3–5 times faster in water than air at the same temperature (Molnar, 1946). The physiological reasons as to why this occurs, and how it can affect performance, will be discussed in the sections below. The implications of training in both cold water and air will also be discussed.

During extreme conditions the body attempts to insulate heat and maintain core temperature as much as possible. Anthropometric characteristics, however, can have a large impact on the rate at which heat loss occurs. The amount of heat loss depends on the surface area to mass ratio (Epstein et al., 1983), which would indicate that taller and lighter individuals are at risk of losing more heat than their shorter and bulkier counterparts. At rest, muscle provides most of the body's insulation (Rennie, 1988), which would suggest those individuals with greater muscle mass would cope with lower temperatures more efficiently. It is in fact subcutaneous adipose tissue that is highly inversely correlated to skin temperature and metabolic rate after exposure to cold air (Smith and Hanna, 1975). Therefore, although contrasting to the ideal somatotype within most athletic sports, a higher percentage of body fat may be preferred with athletes that compete in extreme cold environments.

Rest periods in cold air and water

There are going to be moments, whether before or during exercise, where athletes will be fairly sedentary and may not be able to prevent heat loss. The first defence mechanism is therefore vasoconstriction of the blood vessels, as the body's internal extremities take priority over the skin surface in normal function (Werner and Reents, 1980). It is commonly seen that areas of the body such as the toes, nose and hands are affected first, and feel cold. The general vasoconstriction leads to increased central venous pressure, which leads to a reduced heart rate (Hanna et al., 1975), although a decrease in heart rate is not universally found (Doubt, 1991). In addition to the initial vasoconstriction, metabolic heat is generated through 'pre-shivering', and later shivering (Wagner and Horvath, 1985). Maximal shivering can increase metabolic rate up to four times (Toner and McArdle, 1988) reaching up to 40 per cent VO2 max. This would therefore utilize energy and deplete glycogen stores, so there needs to be consideration of this if our athletes are exposed to extreme cold temperatures. As much insulation as possible should be attempted through clothing, until the body naturally warms up through locomotion and exercise. It is interesting to note that many athletes use an ice bath as a recovery strategy, as prescribed by their coach, although there is a lack of physiological evidence to support this. If they are in there for a prolonged period of time, and the temperature is cold enough, maximal shivering could be elicited, which would be detrimental prior to competition.

It is important to remember for those athletes that may have to compete in open waters of cold temperatures, the effects that cold water can have. When entering the water with an unexpected level of coldness, it could elicit a reflex inspiratory gasp followed by hyperventilation and tachycardia. This can cause a drowning response even in those who are good swimmers (Tipton, 1989). This is known as the cardiorespiratory cold response and can be reduced through repeated exposures prior to the event (Tipton et al., 2000). Therefore, if an athlete is unable to train in cold climates within their training regime, an acclimation process can occur by repeated two-minute exposures. It has been proposed that repeated cold water immersions can last as long as 7–14 months (Tipton et al., 2000). Tipton provides a very good survival manual to avoid this mechanism, and the reader is directed to his work for further information.

Effects of the cold on performance

Water

Exercise in the water at the same temperature as air causes 3–5 times greater heat loss, due to water being 25 times more conductive than air (Smith and Hames, 1962). Even when working at moderate intensities, the metabolic heat generated through swimming is often insufficient to counter the large thermal drain because the heat is lost with constant water moving past the skin (Nadal et al., 1974). Water directly next to the skin when the athlete is still acts as an insulating layer, but when the athlete is moving it becomes less efficient (Toner and McArdle, 1988). One protective way of reducing the effects of heat loss, as touched on earlier, is having a higher fat percentage, which provides a contrast to athletes having an extremely low body fat for high performance. This would only be a consideration for a sport like open water swimming where the risk of an athlete losing heat can be detrimental to performance and health. There is no solution to this physiological response, but the practitioner should be aware and avoid exposing their athletes to the cold if there's no need to.

Air

Exercise in cold environments and the effects it can have on performance, function and well-being depend on three factors: temperature, wind chill, and moisture (rain). For example, the temperature could be moderate but heavy rain would cause the onset of shivering etc. In extreme conditions, exercising at low intensities has the greatest risk, due to athletes possibly not generating enough heat to counter the cold (Weller et al., 1997). It is therefore imperative that suitable clothing is worn for an extra insulating response. However, if this clothing gets wet, its effectiveness is lost and shivering can occur. This has been attributed to cause greater metabolic rate and oxygen consumption (Toner and McArdle, 1988) which would then cause greater glycogen utilization and could start to recruit more type II fibres (Rome et al., 1984), leading to greater fatigue and diminished health.

Moderate and higher intensity exercise (above 70 per cent VO2 max), shows mixed research findings. Studies have demonstrated that below the optimal temperature of 11°C, performance has decreased (Faulkner et al., 1981), whereas other studies have demonstrated no difference in performance below 20°C (Febbraio et al., 1996). There is no known scientific answer as to why these differences occur, but it is suggested that at moderate to high intensity exercise, the extreme cold can have an effect on different individuals. This comes down to a message that is reinforced throughout this book, when trying to reduce injury rates: coaches need to know their athletes individually and how they respond to different environmental conditions. The taller and thinner athletes seem to be greatly affected by the colder environments, although this is a generalization and individual analysis should be completed. It is also important to note that although there is a belief that a cold day can cause greater chance of injury risk in an acute tear of the muscle, there is no evidence to back this up. Just like the lack of scientific evidence within warm-ups, colder muscles aren't necessarily at greater risk of acute strains. In fact, higher levels of fatigue will cause greater chance of injury. However, the muscle should be prepared optimally to perform at high velocities and forces, so if a sprint athlete is competing in extreme cold environments, warm layers should be worn until they feel warm enough during the warm-up to perform some higher velocity drills.

Although the above statements on the effects of the cold seem very physiological at times, the aim is to heighten the practitioner's awareness of the effects of training in the cold. Therefore, simple things like ensuring they have the right clothing, suitable for all weather types, is important. Avoiding unnecessary waiting around in the cold, as the onset of shivering could occur. Also, athletes who compete in open swimming water events could undertake acclimation protocols, to prepare them for the potentially cold temperature of the water. If the effects of the cold become severe, not only is the athlete at risk of decreasing performance, but also at a severe risk of health deterioration, which could be catastrophic in terms of injury and illness such as hypothermia. It is therefore imperative that procedures to avoid this occurring are put in place. Acclimation and acclimatization have been effective in reducing the negative effects of the cold, and could be a possibility when preparing for a particular game or competition. The reader is directed to Nimmo (2004), for an in-depth discussion around exercise in the cold.

IMMUNE FUNCTION AND REDUCING THE RISK OF ILLNESS

After very recently listening to a couple of lectures by Professor Mike Gleeson, who specializes in immunology and its application to sport, I felt it would be essential to relay this within practical terms. Professor Gleeson has a great way of making this topic very simple with clear take-home messages and strategies in an attempt to reduce the chance of illness. It is firstly important to emphasize that attempting to avoid illness is a must as it can cause detraining effects as well as losing valuable time. It could also cause disruption within a team environment if the illness were to spread throughout the team; therefore it is essential that the right precautions are taken. Although it hasn't been proven within the research world, from experience, if illness is neglected and the athlete carries on the normal schedule, there has a high association with injury potential in particular athletes. Within this section, illness refers to an upper respiratory tract infection (URTI).

Effects of exercise on immune function

When looking at exercise in general, the impact it can have on the immune function is quite confusing, and depends on a number of variables. Exercise is demonstrated to have a 'J' shaped association with immune function (Nieman, 1994), which means that there is an optimal duration of exercise that enhances immune function acutely, and if the bout goes over this, then it can suppress the immune system acutely. Exercise, regardless of intensity, up to 90–120 minutes daily has been associated with a 29 per cent decreased risk of a URTI, in comparison with their sedentary counterpart (Matthews et al., 2002). There is conflicting research within endurance training and events, a high volume sport typically associated with immune function. It has been proposed that after a high volume event, such as an ultra-endurance event, athletes have 100–500 per cent increased risk of catching a URTI within the first few hours post-race

(Peters *et al.*, 1993: Peters *et al.*, 1996). However, a more recent study by Ekblom *et al.* (2006), demonstrated no significant relationship between higher volumes of training and URTI caused in endurance athletes leading up to the marathon. What was found, however, was that of those who did report a URTI three weeks prior to the event, almost of all of them suffered post-race, which suggests that training and illness could be an individualized theory itself. It is important, therefore, that those athletes who are more susceptible to URTI, should have their training prescription modified to address this. There is also a suggestion that higher intensity (>75 per cent VO2 max) training can cause greater risk of illness, although this hasn't been demonstrated scientifically, as it would be too hard to control other variables. This would also suggest that athletes shouldn't work above certain thresholds due to an increased chance of illness, which would cause a significant lack of adaptation or detraining. However, correct periodized programmes would have periods where intensity is lower. Although there seems to be some evidence that a high training volume, particularly in an acute bout, can suppress immune function, it is proposed that there is very little difference in immune function between those who train regularly and their sedentary counterparts. This lends itself to the notion that the window post-exercise is most important in avoiding any illness.

The effect exercise has on the immune function has been superficially described here, without delving into any in-depth pathology and physiology. Readers interested in finding out more detail are recommended to read Gleeson's (2007) paper on immune function.

Reducing the spread of URTIs

Aside from reducing the onset of illness, it is now important to provide clear messages that can be implemented within your place of work in an attempt to reduce the recurrence of URTIs. It is firstly important to highlight the importance of good hygiene and reducing the spread of harmful bacteria. Frequent washing of hands, preferably using alcohol-based solutions, would be optimal. In some sports, there is a high culture of shaking hands amongst coaches and athletes; this can then be a breeding ground for bacteria being passed from one person to another. It is also important that all drinks bottles that are reused are cleaned thoroughly and sterilized after use, especially those with glucose-based drinks inside (glucose is an excellent breeding solution for bacteria). This simply reinforces common sense, but good hygiene practice amongst your athletes is essential.

It is also important also that your sports science and medical team have a procedure or protocol for those athletes who do become ill. It is suggested that if an athlete has symptoms above the neck, and has a common cold, they can train as normal (applying caution to the intensity and volume, if the session that was planned was to be really high). If symptoms are below the neck, however, which would mean flu symptoms, severe chest infection, or sickness bug, send them home immediately until their symptoms improve or are gone. Effective communication will be required from physiotherapists and doctors to ensure this decision can be authorized. It is important also that any staff member who becomes seriously ill is removed from the environment also. If an athlete reports illness, then close liaison with the medical and nutritional team should occur to provide any supplementation. Regular vitamins are important to take all around but high doses of vitamin D and C as well as other supplements could reduce the severity and length of illness. There is, however, much research needed within this area although some is reviewed in the last section of this chapter below.

The beginning of this chapter emphasized the importance of sleep on both injury potential and illness. I presented a case that has been found in the practical setting, that those who slept consistently less than 8 hours, had a higher chance of either injury or illness, so its importance is highlighted. An early study in 1997 by Pilcher *et al.*, demonstrated that those who had not only poor quantity but also poor quality of sleep had significantly lower health measures – so for optimal illness avoidance, the quality as well as the quantity is essential to monitor.

Amongst athletes that I currently work with, there is a large percentage of them that need a nutritional intervention in terms of illness. Certainly, all athletes need to be educated on providing their body with substantial amounts of nutrients and minerals, but there is a vitamin in particular that these athletes are deficient in. Due to the lack of sunlight and heat in the winter months (in the United Kingdom in particular), a lot of athletes are vitamin D deficient and need to be supplemented with high doses. The role of vitamin D is essential for strength with the physiological knowledge of the role it plays in muscle function. However, it is proposed to have high effects on illness and bone strength too. Gerdhem *et al.* (2005) provided evidence that lower vitamin D levels within subjects caused greater risk of fractures. It is important to remember that in the summer months there should be enough exposure to sunlight, which would provide enough vitamin D through the skin. It is advisable for athletes to get their bloods tested for vitamin D levels throughout the winter months to see who needs high supplementation.

10 | REHAB FROM AN S&C PERSPECTIVE

This next chapter will prescribe some ideas that strength and conditioning coaches can implement when getting an athlete back to competing in their sport. The aim is not to tread on the toes of the physiotherapist, and will focus on some implementations an S&C coach can do, to enhance the physiological profile of the returning athlete. It will focus more predominately on late stage rehab, and increasing the athletes' physiological qualities (aerobic/anaerobic conditioning), although will begin with some ideas that can reduce the effects of detraining with an immobilized limb. It is essential that a good relationship and understanding is developed with the physiotherapist, so a greater environment and holistic rehab programme is integrated between the two sub-disciplines. Often there is a battle of philosophies and contrasting thoughts between the physio and S&C coach, and in this situation more respect needs to be shown on both sides towards each other's work and knowledge. This cooperation will provide a better rehab programme for the athlete and will ensure that all elements of the rehab programme are included for optimal recovery. It also must be remembered that each injury, with each different player, must be treated individually. This chapter will outline a very vague rehab programme outline that would enhance various physiological qualities; however, the practitioner needs to select what aspects are relevant to their athlete. As frequently mentioned throughout this book, there is a need to individualize training programmes for each athlete, and the same applies for each injury rehab protocol also.

CONTRALATERAL TRAINING

The first pocket of research provides an opportunity for the strength and conditioning coach to perform some work with an injured athlete, even if they have an immobilized limb. It is proposed within literature that training one limb in isolation can make greater strength gains in the untrained limb (Zhou, 2000; Munn et al., 2004). This method is known as contralateral training, or cross-education. A meta-analysis completed by Munn et al. (2005), demonstrated that a strength increase of 8 per cent was found in the control limb that wasn't directly trained, and up to 35 per cent in the limb that was directly trained. This strength increase in the trained limb was so high due to the subjects being fairly untrained in strength qualities, so it would be lower in elite athletes. This provides an essential training technique for avoiding too much detraining and strength loss whilst being injured with an immobilized limb. Without delving into too much detail of muscle physiology, the mechanisms that seem to be responsible are a result of central as opposed to peripheral adaptations (Hellebrandt, 1951). Further, more recent, research reinforces that it is down to greater central adaptations, due to increases in electromyography (EMG) (Ranganathan et al., 2004) and voluntary muscle actions via a twitch interpolation technique involving nerve stimulation (Shima et al., 2002). What is apparent from this technique, however, is that although some strength increase can be made, or at least maintained when an athlete has an immobilized limb, muscular atrophy cannot be avoided during this time period. Therefore, during the rehab programme, a particular focus should be increasing hypertrophy of the muscles required, or those that haven't been used adequately during the immobilization.

MUSCULAR ATROPHY

As discussed in the last section, one of the major detraining effects that occur during long-term injuries is muscular atrophy of the unused limb. It is therefore essential that these particular muscles increase their size, back to normal. Within early stages of rehab, muscular size can be enhanced by effective electrical stimulation to the muscle. Although this technique has been proposed to enhance muscle cross-sectional area, it does not include any neurological improvements associated with strength gains, which limits the method to increasing both size and strength. However, it does provide an effective base for re-activating the muscle fibres and providing some hypertrophic effects.

Following this method, there is a potential technique that can be reintroduced to elicit hypertrophic gains, even if they are not ready for high intensities within the gym. The method is known as 'blood occlusion training'. It is proposed that intensities as low as 20 per cent 1RM, with the addition of vascular occlusion, elicited a significant increase in plasma growth hormone (Takarada et al., 2000a) and muscular hypertrophy over a 16-week period (Takarada et al., 2000b). Takarada et al. (2002) demonstrated further increases in muscular strength and hypertrophy with 50 per cent 1RM and 196 mmHg vascular occlusion pressure. This proposes that muscular hypertrophy increases between 20–60 per cent 1RM and relatively higher volumes with those athletes being reintroduced to strength training, and needing hypertrophy adaptations. Although the pressure of the cuff has been debated within the literature, it is proposed in a paper by Moore et al. (2004) and backed up by my experience that a pressure of 100 mmHg is suitable. This is suggested because if the cuff is too tight, although it restricts blood flow further, the area that has the cuff applied to it has no hypertrophy increase due to blood pooling and muscle damage caused by the cuff. Of course individual variance has to be applied, and if an athlete is significantly larger with greater muscle mass they may be able to tolerate a greater pressure. Even though intensities are relatively low in terms of traditional strength training, they propose an overload to the electrical stimulation and start to acquire some neurological adaptations to strength training.

There are a few explanations that have been proposed to demonstrate why occlusion training can enhance muscular hypertrophy (Loenneke et al., 2010). It is firstly due to the consequence of inhibiting blood to enter the working muscle, limiting the amount of oxygen that is present within the muscle. Therefore, a significant accumulation of metabolic by-products occur, such as hydrogen ions and associated lactate, which provides a greater stimulus for muscle hypertrophy. This in turn provides a significant increase in the m-TOR pathway activation which is essential for adaptations such as muscle hypertrophy. Finally, it was also suggested that even though the intensity was still relatively low, there is a significant increase in both slow twitch and fast twitch muscle fibres, ensuring that a larger percentage of the motor unit is activated and stimulated, which would lead to greater hypertrophy of the muscle over time. It has been found that occlusion training has very little effect on the neuromuscular system and can be repeated the next day if required because muscle damage and neurological fatigue are very low, for example.

INTRODUCING THE ATHLETE TO 'FUNCTIONAL' STRENGTH AND CONDITIONING

It is fundamental that when the athlete can start tolerating more load as they progress through their rehab process, they are integrated back into more traditional strength and conditioning programmes. It is important the athlete doesn't just do their rehab programme before being re-introduced to full training: there needs to be a time where the strength and conditioning coach applies a programme to optimally prepare the athlete to return into training. This section will focus predominately on structural changes and strength work, whereas the physiological conditioning will be discussed in the next section of this chapter.

Maximal strength development was covered in detail at the start of this book, so a brief summary is provided here, along with a continuum an athlete should follow bringing them back to full fitness and readiness for training.

From a loading perspective, the initial stage would be to enhance the mobility and stability of the athlete first, in conjunction with the physiotherapist's work, specifically looking at hip stability, including the correct activation of posterior chain and some introduction to bilateral and unilateral hip hinging ability. Alongside this, knee stability work can be introduced with some single leg exercises around flexion and increasing the depth the athlete can get to and keeping the alignment of the knee joints. A further progression within this stability phase can start to look at low level proprioception balance work, introducing some ankle stability work alongside the ability to control all of the lower limb joints. This phase of stability should not be neglected and provides the opportunity to get the athlete moving well, prior to being put under some higher load. I would then ensure that these types of exercises are still kept within prehab sessions after this phase, and completed in conjunction with the strength work in the gym.

Once the athlete has been cleared they can then start performing some more traditional strength lifts and again, the type of strength work may depend on the type and anatomical region of the injury. The strength work also depends on how much time the athlete has before being integrated into full training also, as this may cause change to various cycles. Having said that, when an injured athlete returns it is a great time to use a more linear periodization model (Siff, 2004). For example, the athlete can do a period of anatomical adaptations, hypertrophy placing the athlete under higher loads, maximal strength work and finally progressing onto the rate of force development (RFD)/explosive power prior to returning to team training. The coach will have to be clever if the rehab time is short as they might have to keep each component cycle short, or start to integrate the strength work alongside with technical/tactical training.

The strength and conditioning coach also needs to consider the effects of concurrent training when developing physiological conditioning parameters alongside various strength qualities. For example, if trying to enhance aerobic qualities on the field, as well as anatomical adaptations/hypertrophy within the gym, the gym session would be preferably done in the afternoon, after an extensive rest period from the morning conditioning. If completed the other way around, the hypertrophic/strength gains will be limited due to a blunting of the m-TOR pathway (Blagrove, 2014). The AMPK pathway that is activated during conditioning work inhibits the m-TOR pathway so adaptation is limited. However, if maximal strength/RFD work is being completed alongside the maximal speed work outside, it would make sense to change the order of sessions and complete the gym session first. On the other hand, there may be times where real focus on the athlete being fresh for maximal speed/agility may take priority, so in this situation the coach needs to optimize the training requirements and targets at that stage of rehab.

PHYSIOLOGICAL CONDITIONING

The injured athlete who has been out for a substantial period of time will require a well-designed physiological training programme, depending on their sport, of course. It is believed by some that within the strength and conditioning field, neglect of the conditioning side occurs, and the strength aspect becomes dominant. However, this has to shift, as an athlete's physiological condition is just as important as their strength profile, although they may cross over. Before the athlete can return to fully loading the joint/muscle, the S&C coach can find alternative exercise methods to create both a central and peripheral adaptation, utilizing the methods that will be discussed in this section. For example, if a runner cannot load the limb through full bodyweight locomotion, they might perform some work in the swimming pool, and on the bike, where the load is taken away or reduced. However, once they can

return to full loaded conditioning, I believe this period gives the opportunity to prescribe a more linear periodized model to enhance the physiological capacity of the athlete. The suggestions and model proposed in this section aim to cover a variety of sports, and the coach should adapt it to what would be relevant to a particular athlete. For example, a sprinter may only need a portion of aerobic conditioning within their rehab in contrast to another athlete, and a distance runner would only work on the aerobic conditioning as it is more specific to their sport.

Stage 1: Aerobic conditioning

When an athlete is returning from long and moderate injuries, it is imperative that they complete some sub-maximal longer steady state training. This is not only for physiological adaptations but also for tolerance of load again post-injury, depending on the anatomical region and type of injury of course. It is well documented that this longer duration sub-maximal type of conditioning elicits greater peripheral adaptations such as a greater transportation and utilization of oxygen from the blood into the muscle (Green et al., 1989; Green et al., 1992). However, due to the high detrained effect of the injured athlete, there will be some central adaptations within this initial period also, such as an increase in blood and plasma volume (Green et al., 1990), lower heart rates at the same levels of work rate (Green et al., 1991), and greater cardiac output and stroke volume (Rowell, 1993). Although some central adaptations would occur, the intensity is arguably too low to elicit any increases in VO2 max (McKenzie et al., 2000). Therefore, some manipulation of intensity would be required to increase VO2 max. However, this stage of sub-maximal longer steady state endurance work is required to provide a physiological foundation of aerobic endurance, before central adaptations are targeted.

Within this end of this phase also, the coach and sports scientist can start to prescribe some intervals around the lactate threshold to improve the ability to buffer lower levels of lactate at the onset of the anaerobic threshold. This would provide a good base for some anaerobic conditioning later on in the rehab programme. It is important that the coach or sports scientist either has data on the athlete's lactate threshold or can predict it using heart rate data and what speed would be required to work at. Weltman et al. (1997) demonstrated that lactate threshold wasn't attained until around 90 per cent heart rate max, and 95 per cent VO2 max. Much depends on the athlete and level of aerobic capacity they have, so ensure you have past data regarding your athlete that you can work off. Increasing the work that can be completed at these intensities would provide essential physiological adaptations at the lactate threshold. It must be remembered that any data collected from the athlete previously prior to training zones may have altered due to the detraining effect during the athlete's injury. Appropriate adjustments need to be made based on the monitoring of the longer steady state sub-maximal work completed in the initial stage of physiological conditioning. It may be important, therefore, to regularly assess the athlete's ability to perform a sub-maximal bout of endurance work whilst they are fit and healthy. The practitioner would then have baseline data that can be compared to the athletes current physiological condition.

The next phase of conditioning would be to perform some high intensity interval training (HIIT), which would require intervals of aerobic bouts between 3 and 5 minutes at approximately 100 per cent VO2 max, or above (supra-maximal), and relatively low recovery times of 1–2 minutes. HIIT has been demonstrated to enhance VO2 max significantly in very short time periods (Hickson et al., 1977). This has been found to maximize central adaptations and the ability to produce greater amounts of oxygen from the central cardiac system (maximizing cardiac output/stroke volume) (Laursen and Jenkins, 2002). Other adaptations include an enhanced oxidative capacity of type II fibres (Billat, 2001) and increased mitochondrial fatty acid oxidation, creating an effective fuel utilization and enhancing economy (Chilibeck et al., 1998). In my opinion, VO2 max is often discredited within certain sports as not being an important physiological variable for performance. Within elite endurance athletes I have to agree with that statement, that other variables will predict performance more accurately (these other variables will be discussed later in this chapter). However, for other sports that are intermittent, place high aerobic emphasis within recovery periods, and aerobic capacity/power is generally not maximized within the athletes, a higher VO2 max would provide numerous benefits. It is firstly proved in numerous studies that the higher the rank of athlete, the higher the VO2 max is (Smith et al., 1992; Gabbet et al., 2007; Van Winckel et al., 2014). Higher aerobic capacities can provide the athlete with greater tolerance to higher training volumes, a lowered risk of injury within later stages of competition, and an acute increase in performance and recovery between intermittent bouts. As alluded to earlier, there are other variables associated with aerobic performance, other than VO2 max, that are important for physiological conditioning, but for many sports that aren't strictly endurance based, VO2 max is an essential physiological component that should not be overlooked.

The next variables associated with increasing aerobic performance come from a long-standing practitioner in Australia, Dan Baker. A well-respected strength and conditioning coach, he has developed his methods of training aerobic capacity within intermittent team sports so the practitioner should apply these techniques if they are appropriate to your athletes. I believe Dan

Baker's approach should be applied after the foundations of peripheral and central adaptations have been set, as described in the sections above.

Baker (2011) uses the term MAS (maximal aerobic speed) and this can be easily calculated by a number of methods. The easiest way is to provide a set distance, 1500–2000 metres has been proposed optimal, and calculate how long it takes the athlete to complete it in. Then divide the distance in metres by the time it takes the athlete to complete in seconds. You can then calculate how much distance the athlete covered per second (this is essential for training prescription later on). For example, an athlete runs 1500 metres in 300 seconds (5 minutes), so the athlete's MAS is 5 m/s.

The rationale behind MAS is based on improving your athlete's ability to run at VO2 max or supra-maximal levels. It can be closely linked to enhancing the velocity the athlete can run at VO2 max (vVO2). In terms of training prescription, Baker (2011) suggests a method known as Eurofit, which I think is a very good method of further enhancing aerobic capacity. It breaks down the aerobic interval (3–5 mins) and splits it into further aerobic intervals of 15 seconds on and 15 seconds off. This method should be completed at 110 per cent, progressing onto 120 per cent MAS level. For example, taking the athlete with a 5 m/s MAS, 110 per cent would equal 5.5 m/s for 15 seconds' work. This would equal a total distance within each 15-second interval of 82.5 metres. This athlete would be a fairly well-trained endurance athlete and lower scores would be expected, especially within team sports. It is essential that further physiological monitoring is done to ensure the athlete is still working within aerobic zones (utilizing HR/lactate monitoring tools). If you have any athlete who might be an outlier, e.g. one who is very aerobic-based with little difference in maximal speed ability (a plodder), or one who is explosive but has

extremely low aerobic capacity, then there is a further method you can use to calculate their Eurofit intensity more accurately. Instead of using 120 per cent MAS, you can use 100 per cent MAS + 30 per cent anaerobic speed reserve (ASR). ASR is calculated by taking your MAS score away from the athlete's maximum velocity you can calculate from a timed sprint with flying start so the athlete is in top velocity phase, or measured during the top speed phase using GPS devices etc.

A further progression from Dan Baker's Eurofit concept is the method of Tabata et al. (1996) where the same measures of intensity can be used from Dan Baker's methods (120 per cent MAS or 100 per cent MAS + 30 per cent ASR) and applied to the time intervals of 20 seconds on and 10 seconds off. This applies the basic principles of training, applying an overload of relative volume of work within the same overall volume of work. Furthermore, the work volume within 4 × 4 minutes of Eurofit would be half of the time (8 minutes/480 seconds) whereas the Tabata method would elicit over 10½ minutes of work (640 seconds). Baker proposes that Tabata is used with one or two turns in and therefore a significant decrease in distance is required to accommodate for the turns. In my opinion, especially with rehab protocols, is there a need to apply turns in? It could be more specific to the sport, however: if maximal gains in aerobic ability are required, then use the straight line running for 20 seconds at 110/120 per cent MAS, as this will optimize the physiological adaptation required. Too many coaches become hooked on specificity; plan what physiological adaptation you want, and the best way to develop it.

It must be remembered that within all of the aerobic methods described in this last section it is down to the coach how certain variables are progressed. With longer steady state sub-maximal exercise the best way to overload is through volume, and when a particular volume or duration of exercise can be completed, it would be advisable to move onto higher intensity intervals. HIIT can provide many methods for progression: increasing volume of the interval (3 to 5 minutes over a period of time); increasing the number of sets completed (3 to 6 sets); or ensuring the athlete can increase the intensity and cover more distance in the same time frame. The coach, therefore, needs to assess the time frame they have for their athlete, and provide a plan with good progression of physiological components. As well as the benefits of aerobic conditioning, it is essential that within many sports that are intermittent, their anaerobic abilities are enhanced as well during the rehab process. The next section of this chapter will therefore focus on my experiences and ideas around developing anaerobic variables within an athlete's rehab.

Although each phase might focus on a different area of aerobic conditioning, don't be afraid to maintain other qualities within your programmes. For example, a sub-maximal longer steady state run might still be completed once a week to maintain the peripheral adaptations gained. Endurance athletes will do this all year round for this reason and to enhance running economy/efficiency.

Stage 2: Anaerobic conditioning

This next section depicts my experiences amongst anaerobic conditioning in sports that are intermittent, ensuring the athlete can handle the repeated anaerobic bouts of exercise, before returning to competition. This phase is obviously very important, and depends largely on the athlete's aerobic abilities. If an athlete has a higher aerobic base they will be able to recover faster between high intensity bouts, due to faster replenishment of ATP/PCr stores and removal of acidic by-products (Tomlin and Wenger, 2001). This justifies my rationale to structure the rehab conditioning in a linear periodized method, where aerobic conditioning is prescribed prior to anaerobic conditioning as it precedes the other quality, as opposed to a more undulated method you might use with a fully fit athlete in season.

Following the natural linear model it would make sense to start with some higher volume anaerobic conditioning, known as lactate stacking. Although it has been established that lactate may not be the primal reason for fatigue, it has an extremely strong correlation with other acidic by-products such as hydrogen ions, which would cause fatigue levels. Blood lactate levels therefore can be an accurate measure and indicator of high intensity fatigue. Within this phase, maximal bouts of 45–90 seconds are required with relatively short recovery periods. A huge difference between aerobic and anaerobic conditioning is that within anaerobic work, the intervals are always maximal, or close to it. Aerobic intervals can vary as to whether they are maximal or not, as it is essential that at times the anaerobic energy stores are not used. Work:rest ratios within this lactate stacking method of 1:2 and 1:1 would provide an effective stimulus for the athlete to have to buffer required acidic by-products efficiently to enhance performance. It must be remembered that although this conditioning is not specific to that performed in the athlete's sport (unless they are a 400 metre runner or equivalent in a different sport), overload within all of these training methods is essential, to maximize that particular physiological quality. Too many coaches worry about making everything sport specific. At times specificity is essential but for enhancing physiological qualities, the coach needs to assess the best way to do that in isolation, which will have a significant and positive effect within that athlete's post-rehab sporting performance.

The next phase of the rehab now reduces the volume even more, and increases the intensity of the work. Repeated sprint ability is a key physical quality that determines successful performance in many intermittent sports (Girard *et al.*, 2011). As mentioned before, however, it is largely dependent on the athlete's aerobic abilities, therefore it is strongly recommended that for greater RSA and lower injury rates, that a higher aerobic base is established. When designing RSA programmes it is essential that the athlete is exposed to a variety of distances covered (10–50 metres), with a variety of work:rest ratios, and a variety of interval structure (i.e. with changes of direction/linear etc.). I would urge the practitioner to start off with the overload principle in mind, and as the athlete gets to the end stages of the phase, start to mimic the sporting demands more closely. There are lots of research papers out there that show time–motion analysis of each sport and would suggest what each position performed in that study. However, coaches need to be going beyond using the data of someone else's athletes, and should refer to the sports science data available on your athlete to create the most position-specific physiological rehab programme. Close liaison with the sports scientist and GPS data is required to create this programme and be more effective. This leaves the athlete in a good position for them to return to the most specific conditioning they could do, and that is the sport training itself.

Stage 3: Sport-specific return to training

The next phase then sees the athlete returning to team training for their sport-specific conditioning. Small-sided games in many sports have been used for a number of years now to elicit a training and physiological adaptation. Raymond Verheijen within soccer has created a periodized SSG structure that manipulates the dimension of the pitch, team numbers and duration of SSG to provide a different physiological adaptation. This technique is also evident from a Portuguese tactical periodization model in the newly published book by Van Winckel *et al.* (2014). When monitoring these conditioning games within training, GPS can become a very productive tool. Within small-dimension games an overload of acceleration and decelerations would be the emphasis, whereas in larger games greater distance covered and higher metabolic load would be a desired outcome of the session. The aim would be to work supra-maximal to that of a game within a certain time period. So it is relatively higher intensity and overloaded in relation to a game, with a significantly lower overall volume. Although SSGs are an effective tool used for conditioning athletes with an integrated technical/tactical component, it is suggested that some supplementary conditioning is still needed for central adaptations (Buchheit and Laursen, 2013). SSGs predominantly elicit peripheral adaptations so some higher intensity central work is required to maintain or overload that physiological quality, depending on the aims of that phase.

This conditioning periodization also needs to consider the development of movement patterns such as maximal speed and agility tasks, which need to be completed in conjunction with the S&C work to optimize the athlete's rehab. Speed preparation work at 60 per cent max speed should be implemented when the physio and practitioner think the athlete can tolerate this intensity, and progressed accordingly to develop maximal speed/agility patterns, closer to the end stage rehab process and the return to training. Remember: although you can develop maximal speed, and enhance agility in isolation with a variety of closed/open chain and reactive drills, the sporting training itself will be the best rehab and development of specific speed/agility.

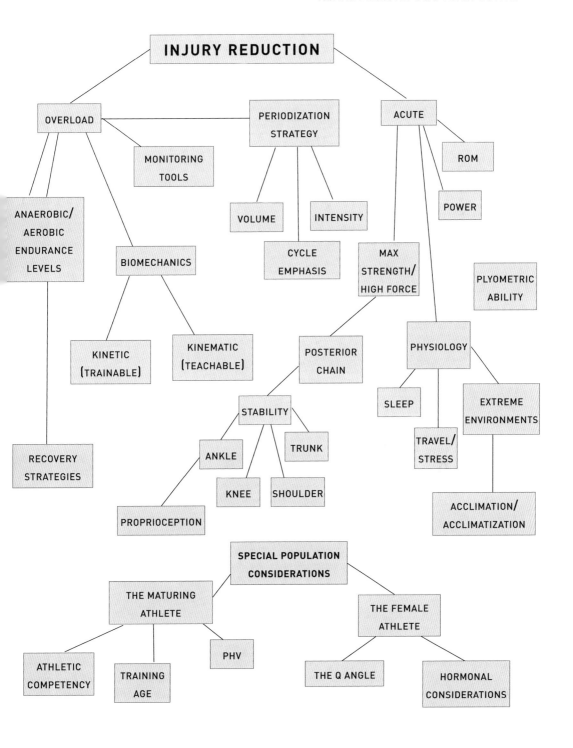

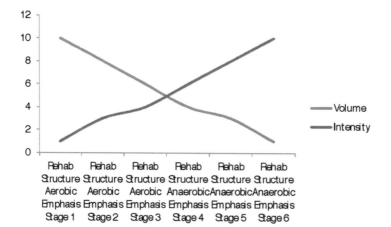

The preferred linear periodized structure in the physiological conditioning aspect of rehabilitating a moderate- to long-term injured athlete.

SUMMARY

The graph above represents the linear periodized structure that is preferred in the physiological conditioning aspect of rehabilitating a moderate- to long-term injured athlete. The volume and intensity scale figures are arbitrary and are used to represent the concept as opposed to giving specific figures. As is evident, the programme starts with aerobic emphasis and higher volume work that would elicit central and peripheral adaptations through the different methods discussed. As the emphasis becomes anaerobic the volume reduces and intensity of work increases and so on. In my opinion, rehab should be performed in more of a linear structure to saturate a physical quality before progressing onto a different stimulus. It also introduces the athlete to gradual increases in intensity as the rehab progresses further.

What is important is the consideration of concurrent training during the rehab process. It is recommended that the athlete should follow a similar linear model of gym-based work around hypertrophy, strength and power. According to Blagrove (2014), this needs to be a consideration to ensure maximal adaptation occurs and there isn't a blocking of progression of certain qualities due to the programme. Therefore, if the volume is high within the conditioning element, the strength work volume should be lower, and performed significantly after the conditioning work, to avoid the m-TOR pathway being blocked. The coach needs to be creative and construct a programme with all the elements required together, to optimize adaptation with all elements required.

One thing that needs to be mentioned is the likelihood of an athlete breaking down. At times, regardless of how well designed a rehab programme is, there is always a chance an athlete will break down at some stage. At first, I would make myself responsible for that and question my programming abilities. However, as a practitioner you must understand that this could happen with any athlete, at any particular stage if they have had a long-term injury. Of course we want to avoid this, but in the rehab stage, the athlete is bound to feel some niggles or break down if they are pushed too much. Of course the athlete has to be pushed for maximal adaptation, so a balance needs to be established. The more experience you gain as a coach, writing and performing rehab programmes, the better you'll be able to judge it; however, every athlete is different and will be able tolerate different amounts of load.

11 APPLIED CASE STUDY: PUTTING THEORY INTO PRACTICE

This final chapter of the book provides an individual case study of an athlete with whom I am currently working to enhance the time spent training, to reduce injury risk, and to increase his physical performance. It is my aim to incorporate as many of the topics discussed within this book as possible, to apply the theory into a real-life scenario.

BACKGROUND INFORMATION

The subject is an elite youth footballer, who plays for a premiership football club and has been in the academy for eight years. He has received strength and conditioning support for the last two years, learning basic gym competencies and on-field technical locomotive skills. His physiological testing profile will be outlined below to provide an overview of the athlete in both performance and injury prevention tests. He has suffered previously with lateral knee pain and adductor overload injuries, which has caused him to miss training and games at times.

Performance tests

Aerobic capacity
1600 metre run: 5'22''
YoYo Intermittent Recovery Test 2: Level 16

Maximal strength
1RM half squat: 135kg
Normalized half squat (kg/kg–bw): 1.92

Speed/acceleration
10m sprint: 1.75
30m sprint: 4.45

Power/jump
Squat jump: 32cm
Counter-movement jump: 35cm

Injury prevention tests

Overhead squat
Scored a 1 (poor mover), with extreme tightness and lack of ROM from all joints (ankle, hip and thoracic). This was reinforced with poor ROM identified in further tests performed by the physiotherapist.

Single leg squat
Identified high amounts of knee valgus indicating poor ankle mobility and/or weak

hip abductors which was proven further with isometric dynamometer tests of the hip abductors. He also demonstrated an internal trunk rotation which suggested weak external obliques and a dysfunctional anterior sling.

Knee to wall (ankle mobility)
Right: 3cm
Left: 2cm

Although some of the above performance tests may be criticized for not directly assessing the physiological quality, the reader must understand that within an applied setting it is often difficult to have access to a laboratory, so tests that can be done with very limited resources are preferred. Of course in an ideal world a VO2 max test would be performed; however, the 1600 metre is selected to provide a rough outline of the athlete's aerobic ability. The 1600 metre run is also done to assess the athlete's maximal aerobic speed (Baker, 2011) as discussed in the rehab chapter. As well as the 1600 metre test we conducted the YoYo IRT2, which is obviously more specific to football, and assesses both aerobic and anaerobic endurance qualities. It was found that the 1600 metre run had a very strong correlation with the YoYo IRT2 test within this cohort. The YoYo IRT2 also provides us with an estimated VO2 max of 66ml/kg, which again correlates very strongly with previous internal research.

Outcome

It is clear from the performance tests that this athlete, although he is very good aerobically for a football player, is very poor within high force/power/velocity tasks. He has also demonstrated extremely poor single leg stability and mobility from the injury prevention tests/screening procedures. It is therefore apparent that this athlete needs much S&C work to enhance his athletic performance and reduce the risk of injury.

PROGRAMME PRESCRIPTION AND PROBLEMS

As a traditional strength and conditioning coach, I would always endorse strength training, and squatting would normally be a prioritized exercise. However, in this particular case, the traditional strength training exercises initially proved detrimental to this athlete's development. Due to this athlete's lack of mobility, particularly ankle mobility, when he squats with heavy load (relatively) he compensates the lack of ankle mobility with high amounts of internal rotation of the femur and knee valgus. This poor biomechanical compensation and dysfunction shown in strength training movements is occurring in every sporting action as well, which is why squatting is actually adding load to particular joints and muscles that are already being overloaded in the sport, enhancing his risk of injury.

In this case it is therefore important that the dysfunctions are fixed before any performance enhancement exercises such as squatting are put back into this athlete's programme. The message to the practising strength and conditioning coach is clear: though the importance of getting athletes stronger is frequently stated (which is true and this principle underpins many performance variables and injury resistance), as a coach you need to know individual players and you must be adaptable. In this case taking squatting out of his programme and fixing the issues will be more beneficial to his athletic development. After these dysfunctions are then improved, he can perform certain movements efficiently and avoid overload injuries, eradicating poor limb alignment and compensation at particular joints.

The reason why I selected this particular case study was to highlight that traditional strength doesn't always provide the solution, although its benefits are huge with the functional athlete with good mobility. There are times when it might add additional load to poor mobility and motor patterns, which need to be addressed prior to heavier strength training. This method combines the traditional strength method with corrective exercise and amongst certain athletes (such as footballers) can provide effective foundations for heavier and more advanced strength training. As well as poor ankle mobility, as noted earlier, poor hip abductor strength is causing this athlete high amounts of internal rotation and knee valgus. These are therefore the main aims of the initial training programme, as outlined below.

PROGRAMME 1 (8 WEEKS)

Exercise	Sets	Reps
Glute superset (bridges, band walks, resisted abduction)	2	15
Single leg sit down (partial depth)	2	6
Step up/reverse step down	2	6
Knee to wall	3	10 sec
Overhead squat (technical)	3	6
Side plank	2	30 sec (each side)
Leg press	3	6
Nordics	3	6

This first programme provides a very cautious approach, particularly for a traditional S&C coach. It aims to improve the dysfunctions found in the screening process, in particular the weak hip abductors and gluteal strength, by isolating the various muscle groups and working them through single leg exercises. Ankle mobility needs to be increased prior to patterning it into an overhead squat. Other ankle mobility work would be done with the physiotherapist to improve this further. Also,

internal/external obliques were targeted by increasing the stiffness of that area. Furthermore, before the traditional strength and conditioning coach laughs at the final exercise, 'leg press', there is a scientific and practice-based evidence behind it, as I shall demonstrate.

Within this initial programme, the aim is to avoid any deep flexion patterns where this athlete is highly compensating to reach these levels. Therefore, the leg press exercise provides the athlete with a chance to increase the force they can produce in a triple extension pattern, in a greater range without compensating, albeit in fixed, stable and assisted context. I am not for one minute suggesting that machine weights are better than free weights, and the industry has moved on from these older beliefs; however, it can add value to an individual's programme if used for the right reason. This is also the reason why the athlete is only partially squatting within the single leg exercises. Due to poor mobility and stability, going into any more flexion would only cause him to compensate into poor motor patterns that we were trying to avoid. Of course the athlete will be going into these poor motor patterns within sporting training, so adding more load to these motor patterns would have increased the risk of injury.

Note the test results below, after the athlete had completed the initial programme. Within the performance tests, although the focus hasn't been on increasing these parameters directly, the current programme along with the sport-specific football training, has elicited some improvement in all of these parameters below. It must be noted, however, that the aim of this programme wasn't to increase physical performance, but reduce injury risk. Within these injury reduction exercises you can see there is a vast improvement in his mobility within certain joints and movements – a better platform for some more advanced training in the gym.

Performance tests

Aerobic capacity
1600 metre run: 5'18''
YoYo Intermittent Recovery Test 2: Level 16

Maximal strength
1RM half squat: 140kg
Normalized half squat (kg/kg–bw): 1.99

Speed/acceleration
10m sprint: 1.74
30m sprint: 4.42

Power/jump
Squat jump: 37cm
Counter-movement jump: 43cm

Injury prevention tests

Overhead squat

Scored a 2 (average mover), and demonstrated improvements in range and getting to parallel without any compensation. Visually more mobility around the ankle joint, enabling greater dorsiflexion.

Single leg squat
Visual tracking of the knee showed an improvement, going into less valgus on the descent to control the joint stability. Looked very strong within the partial range he had been training in and started to compensate once he went past this with some knee valgus and trunk external rotation.

Knee to wall (ankle mobility)
Right: 6cm
Left: 7cm

PROGRAMME 2 (6 WEEKS)

Exercise	Sets	Reps
Glute superset (single leg bridges, band walks, resisted abduction)	2	15
Single leg sit down (parallel squatting)	2	6
Step up/reverse step down (greater range)	26	
Knee to wall	3	10 sec
Overhead squat (technical)	3	6 sec
Front plank and side plank	2	45 sec (each side)
Box squat (parallel)	3	6
Split squats	3	6
RDL	3	6

The next programme prescription, at first glance, doesn't seem too different from the previous programme, as all the prehab/dysfunction exercises still remain and seem to be the main focus of the session. As a department, we wanted to continue the good work and progression we had made with this athlete. Therefore, the programme aims to enhance these qualities further whilst introducing some more 'functional' free weight exercises as his body can now do so without compensating and going into poor motor patterns. Results are seen below from the end of this six-week programme. Aside from this the physiotherapist enhanced and progressed ankle mobility work.

Performance tests

Aerobic capacity
1600 metre run: 5'19''
YoYo Intermittent Recovery Test 2: Level 16

Maximal strength
1RM half squat: 150kg
Normalized half squat (kg/kg–bw): 2.13

Speed/Acceleration
10m sprint: 1.72
30m sprint: 4.41

Power/Jump
Squat jump: 40cm
Counter-movement jump: 45cm

Injury prevention tests

Overhead squat
Scored a 2/3 (average/good mover), and demonstrated further improvements in range and getting just below parallel without any compensation. Visually looked more mobile around the ankle joint, enabling greater dorsiflexion.

Single Leg Squat
Improved again the visual tracking of the knee, going into less valgus on the descent to control the joint stability. Looked very strong within the range to parallel he had been training. Compensated slightly below parallel, although had the range and strength to perform a bodyweight single squat below parallel, which he couldn't do before.

Knee to wall (ankle mobility)
Right: 10cm
Left: 12cm

PROGRAMME 3 (6 WEEKS)

Session 1

Exercise	Sets	Reps
Weighted glute bridges	2	10
Knee to wall	2	10 secs
Box jumps	3	4
Front squats	3	6
Lunges	3	6
Single leg RDL	3	6

Session 2

Exercise	Sets	Reps
Single leg glute bridges	2	10
Knee to wall	2	10 secs
Single leg box jumps	3	4
Deadlifts	3	6
Step-ups (large ROM)	3	6
Nordics (progress to weighted Nordics)	3	6

Phase 3 demonstrated less emphasis on the dysfunctions and prehab as the athlete was in an adequate place regarding mobility/stability and the focus now was to enhance these qualities within the performance exercises. More traditional strength training exercises were prescribed along with some introductory concentric dominant plyometric exercises to focus more on increasing higher force/velocity characteristics. See results below after this final phase.

131

Performance tests

Aerobic capacity
1600 metre run: 5'26''
YoYo Intermittent Recovery Test 2: Level 16

Maximal strength
1RM half squat: 160kg
Normalized half squat (kg/kg–bw): 2.27

Speed/acceleration
10m sprint: 1.68
30m sprint: 4.25

Power/jump
Squat jump: 42cm
Counter-movement jump: 49cm

Injury prevention tests

Overhead squat
Scored a 3 (good mover), demonstrated good range with very little compensation at any particular joints etc.

Single leg squat
Demonstrated good single leg squatting (below parallel), with very little compensation again from joints etc.

Knee to wall (ankle mobility)
Right: 12cm
Left: 13cm

As evident above, even when the programme shifts to a more functional strength and conditioning programme, this can still enhance ROM and stability, if the athlete has relatively good foundations to begin with. The decision to fix these dysfunctions first, before prescribing what I would call a functional performance enhancement programme, seemed to be effective with this individual. From a performance perspective, strength/power/speed scores all increased/decreased accordingly after this programme as you would expect with such a stimulus applied. As you can see, the athlete's aerobic capacity level decreased, due to a heavy match period the phase before, so on field activity was modified and reduced, which meant more focus could be applied to characteristics in the gym etc.

Summary

This case study has provided a good example of how an extremely individualized approach needs to be taken with each athlete; even if they have a similar training history to their team mates, their genetic and pre-disposed biomechanical qualities could dictate their initial motor patterns etc. It is therefore down to the practitioner to ensure that the athlete is prescribed a programme that looks at their holistic physical development. Furthermore, although getting an athlete to squat/jump/Olympic lift will be extremely beneficial and will provide improvements in strength/power, which in turn will enhance speed and so on, is it doing so at a heightened risk of injury due to poor movement patterns. Therefore, attempt to correct the dysfunctions and be creative in getting a physical improvement, before advancing them on.

This particular athlete was extremely poor, and did not reflect the squad average; the majority of athletes could squat with little compensation, but it was important to highlight a case that required lateral thinking from the practitioner, implementing strategies that hadn't necessarily been taught.

REFERENCES

CHAPTER 1 – THE IMPORTANCE OF MAXIMAL STRENGTH

Baechle, T.R., and Earle, R.W. (2000). *Essentials of Strength and Conditioning Training.* Human Kinetics: Champaign, IL.

Behm, D.G., and Andersen, K.G. (2006). 'The role of instability within resistance training.' *Journal of Strength and Conditioning Research.* 20, 716–722.

Bodreau, S.N., Dwyer, M.K., Mattacola, C.G. *et al.* (2005). 'Hip muscle activation during the lunge, single leg squat and step and over exercises.' *Journal of Sport Rehabilitation.* 18, 91–103.

Caterisano, A.R.F., Moss, T.K., Pellinger, K. *et al.* (2002). 'The effects of back squat depth on the EMG activity of four superficial hip and thigh muscles.' *Journal of Strength and Conditioning Research.* 16, 428–432.

Cook, G., Burton, L., Hoogenboom, B. (2006). 'Pre-participation screening: The use of fundamental movement as an assessment of function, Part 1.' *Northern American Journal of Sports Physical Therapy.* 2, 62–72.

Croisier, J.L., Ganteaume, P.T., Binet, J. *et al.* (2008). 'Strength Imbalances and prevention of hamstring injury in professional soccer players.' *American Journal of Sports Medicine.* 36, 1469–1475.

Davidsen, P.K., Gallagher, I.J., Hartman, J.W. *et al.* (2011). 'High responders to resistance exercise training demonstrate differential regulation of skeletal muscle microRNA expression'. *Journal of Applied Physiology.* 100, 309–317.

Escamilla, R.F. (2001). 'Knee biomechanics of the dynamic squat exercise.' *Medicine and Science in Sport and Exercise.* 29, 532–539.

Hill, A.V. (1953). 'The mechanics of active muscle.' *Proceedings of the Royal Society, B.* 141, 104–117.

Huxley, A.F. (1957). 'Muscle structure and theories of contraction.' *Progress in Biophysics and Biophysical Chemistry.* 7, 255–318.

Isear, J.A., Erickson, J.C., and Worrel, T.W. (1999). 'EMG analysis of lower extremity muscle recruitment patterns during an unloaded squat.' *Medicine and Science in Sport and Exercise.* 29, 532–539.

Olsen, O.E., Mykleburst, G., Engerbresten, L. *et al.* (2005). 'Exercises to prevent lower limb injuries in youth sports.' *British Medical Journal.* 330, 1–7.

Roig, M., O'Brien, K., and Kirk, G. (2009). 'The effects of eccentric versus concentric resistance training on muscle strength and mass in healthy adults: A systematic review with meta-analysis.'

Siff, M. (2003). *Supertraining.* Supertraining Institute: Denver.

Stafford, I. (2005). 'Coaching for long term athlete development: To improve participation and performance in sport.'

Stone, M.H., O'Bryant, H.S., Schilling, B.K. *et al.* (1999a). 'Periodization: Effects of manipulating volume and intensity, Part 1.' *National Strength and Conditioning Association.* 21, 56–62.

Stone, M.H., O'Bryant, H.S., Schilling, B.K *et al.* (1999b). 'Periodization: Effects of manipulating volume and intensity, Part 2.' *National Strength and Conditioning Association.* 21, 54–60.

CHAPTER 2 – MANAGING RECOVERY AND AVOIDING OVERTRAINING

Aubert, A.E., Seps, B., and Beckers, F.C. (2003). 'Heart rate variability in athletes.' *Sports Medicine.* 33, 889–919.

Baechle, T.R., and Earle, R.W. (2000). *Essentials of Strength and Conditioning Training.* Human Kinetics: Champaigne, IL.

Baker, D. (2011). 'Recent trends in high intensity aerobic training for field sports.' *UKSCA Journal.* 22, 3–7.

Blagrove, R. (2014). 'Minimising the interference effect during programmes of concurrent strength and endurance training, Part 2: Progamming recommendations.' *UKSCA Journal.* 32, 13–20.

Bleakley, C.M., and Davison, G.W. (2010). 'What is the biochemical and physiological rationale for using cold water immersion in sport recovery? A systematic review.' *British Journal of Sports Medicine.* 44, 179–187.

Blennerhassett, M.G., Vignjevic, P., Vermillion, P. *et al.* (1992). 'Inflammation causes hyperplasia and hypertrophy in smooth muscle of rat small intestine.' *American Journal of Physiology.* 262, 1041–1046.

Buchheit, M., Mendez-Villanueva, A.,

Simpson, B.M. *et al.* (2010). 'Repeated sprint sequences during youth soccer matches.' *Journal of Sports Medicine.* 10, 1–8.

Budgett, R. (2000). 'Overtraining and chronic fatigue: the unexplained under-performance syndrome (UPS)' *International SportsMed Journal* 1, 12-19.

Burke, E.R., and Ekblom, B. (1982). 'Influence of fluid ingestion and dehydration on precision and endurance in tennis.' *Athletic Training.* 275–277.

Chadd, N. (2010). 'An approach to the periodisation of training during the in season for team sports.' *UKSCA Journal.* 21, 17–21.

Choi, D., Cole, K.J., Goodpaster, B.H. *et al.* (1994). 'Effects of passive and active recovery on the resynthesis of muscle glycogen.' *Medicine and Science in Sport and Exercise.* 28, 1327–1330.

Comfort, P., Stewart, A., Bloom, L. *et al.* (2014). 'Relationship between strength, sprint, and jump performance in well trained youth soccer players.' *Journal of Strength and Conditioning Research.* 28, 173–177.

Coutts, A.J., Rampi'nini, E., Marcora, S.M. (2009). 'Heart rate and blood lactate correlates with perceived exertion during small sided soccer games.' *Journal of Science and Medicine in Sport.* 12, 79–84.

Coyle, E.F. (1991). 'Timing and method of increased carbohydrate intake to cope with heavy training, competition and recovery.' *Journal of Sports Sciences.* 9, 29–52.

Dohm, G.L. (2002). 'Exercise effects on muscle insulin signalling and action: Regulation of skeletal muscle GLUT–4 expression by exercise.' *Journal of Applied Physiology.* 93, 782–787.

Dunbar, C.C., Robertson, R.J., Baun, R., *et al.* (1992). 'The validity of regulating exercise intensity by ratings of perceived exertion.' *Medicine and Science in Sport and Exercise.* 24, 94–99.

Ekblom, B. (1986). 'Applied physiology of soccer.' *Sports Medicine.* 3, 50–60.

Ekblom, B. (2002). *Assessment of fitness and player profiles.* International Football and Sports Medicine Conference: Beverley Hills, CA. 22–24 March.

Flanagan, E.P., and Comyns, T.M. (2008). 'The use of contact times and the reactive strength index to optimize the fast stretch-shortening cycle training.' *National Strength and Conditioning Association.* 30, 32–38.

Gaesser, G.A., and Brooks, G.A. (1984). 'Metabolic bases of excess post-exercise oxygen consumption: A review.' *Medicine and Science in Sport and Exercise.* 16, 29–43.

Gleeson, T.T. (1982). 'Lactate and glycogen metabolism during and after exercise in the lizard Sceloporus occidentalis.' *Journal of Comparative Physiology.* 147, 79–84.

Haff, G. (2004a). Roundtable discussion. 'Periodization of training, Part 1.' *National Strength and Conditioning Association.* 26, 50–69.

Haff, G. (2004b). Roundtable discussion. 'Periodization of training, Part 2.' *National Strength and Conditioning Association.* 26, 56–70.

Haff, G. (2010). 'Quantifying workloads in resistance training: A brief review.' *UKSCA Journal.* 19, 31–40.

Harvat, M., Ramsey, V., Franklin, C. *et al.* (2003). 'A method for predicting maximal strength in collegiate women athletes.' *Journal of Strength and Conditioning Research.* 17, 289–304.

Hemmings, B. Smith, M., Craydon, J. et al. (2000). 'Effects of massage on physiological restoration, perceived recovery, and repeated sprint performance', *British Journal of Sports Medicine,* 34, 109-114.

Hopkins, W.G. (2004). *A review on statistics.*

Ivy, J.L., Katz, A.L., Cutler, C.L., *et al.* (1988). 'Muscle glycogen synthesis after exercise: Effect of time of carbohydrate ingestion.' *Journal of Applied Physiology.* 65, 2018–2023.

Kindermann, W., Simon, G., and Keul, J. (1979). 'The significance of the aerobic–anaerobic transition for the determining of work load intensities during endurance training.' *European Journal of Applied Physiology.* 42, 25–34.

Lloyd, R.S., Oliver, J.L., Hughes, M.G. *et al.* (2009). 'Reliability and validity of field based measures of leg stiffness and reactive strength index in youths.' *Journal of Sports Sciences.* 27, 1565–1573.

Maughan, R.J., and Shirreffs, S.M. (2000). 'Rehydration and recovery after exercise.' *Science and Sports.* 19, 234–238.

Oliver, J., Armstrong, N., and Williams, C. (2008). 'Changes in jump performance and muscle activity following soccer specific exercise.' *Journal of Sports Sciences.* 26, 141–148.

Plisk, S., and Stone, M.H. (2003). Periodization strategies. *National Strength and Conditioning Association.*

Ramussen, B.B., Tipton, K.D., Miller, S.L. *et al.* (2000). 'An oral essential amino acid carbohydrate supplement enhances muscle protein anabolism after resistance exercise.' *Journal of Applied Physiology.* 88, 386–392.

Reilly, T., and Ekblom, B. (2005). 'The use of recovery methods post-exercise.' *Journal of Sports Sciences.* 23, 619–627.

Reilly, T., and Rigby, M. (2002). 'Effect of an active warm-down following competitive soccer.' In: *Science and Football IV.* London:

Routledge.

Ryan, A. (1980). 'The neglected art of massage.' *Physician and Sports Medicine.* 8, 25.

Siff, M. (2003). *Supertraining.* Supertraining Institute: Denver.

Stamford, B. (1985). 'Massage for athletes.' *Physician and Sports Medicine.* 13, 176.

Stone, M.H., O'Bryant, H.S., Schilling, B.K. *et al.* (1999a). 'Periodization: Effects of manipulating volume and intensity, Part 1.' *National Strength and Conditioning Association.* 21, 56–62.

Stone, M.H., O'Bryant, H.S., Schilling, B.K. *et al.* (1999b). 'Periodization: Effects of manipulating volume and intensity, Part 2.' *National Strength and Conditioning Association.* 21, 54–60.

Tabata, I., Nishimura, K., Kouzaki, M., *et al.* (1996). 'Effects of moderate intensity and high intensity intermittent training on anaerobic capacity and VO2 max.' *Medicine and Science in Sport and Exercise.* 28, 1327–1330.

Tan, B. (1999). 'Manipulating resistance training program variables to optimize maximum strength in men: A review.' *Journal of Strength and Conditioning Research.* 13, 289–304.

Tipton, K.D., and Wolfe, R.R. (2001). 'Exercise, protein metabolism and muscle growth.' *International Journal of Sports Nutrition and Exercise Metabolism.* 11, 109–112.

Turner, A., Stewart, P., Bishop, C. *et al.* (2014). 'Avoiding overtraining and monitor fatigue.' *UKSCA Journal.* 23, 19–25.

Van Winckel, J., Helsen, W., McMillan, K. *et al.* (2014). *Fitness in Soccer: The Science and Practical Application.*

White, G.E., and Wells, G.D. (2013). 'Cold water immersion and other forms of cryotherapy: Physiological changes potentially affecting recovery from high intensity exercise.' *Exercise Physiology and Medicine.* 26, 2–6.

Ylinen, J., and Cash, M. (1988). *Sports Massage.* London: Stanley Paul.

CHAPTER 3 – RANGE OF MOVEMENT AND CORRECTIVE EXERCISE

Behm, D.G., and Chaouachi, A. (2011). 'A review of the acute effects of static and dynamic stretching on performance.' *European Journal of Applied Physiology.* 111, 2633–2651.

Clark, M., & Lucett, S. (2010). *NASM Essentials of Corrective Exercise Training.*

Cleak, M.J., and Eston, R.G. (1992). 'Delayed onset of muscle soreness; mechanisms and management.' *Journal of Sports Sciences.* 10, 31–36.

Cook, G. (2010). *Movement: Functional movement systems – screening, assessing, corrective strategies.* On Target Publications: USA.

Dumke, C.L., Pffafenroth, C.M., McBride, J.M. *et al.* (2010). 'Relationship between muscle strength, power and stiffness and running economy in trained male runners.' *International Journal of Sports Physiology and Performance.* 5, 249–261.

Jeffreys, I. (2007). 'Warm up revisited – the 'ramp' method of optimising performance preparation.' *UKSCA Journal.* 6, 15–19.

Kibler, B.W., Chandler, T.J., Livingston, B.P. *et al.* (1996). 'Shoulder range of motion in elite tennis players: Effects of age and years of tournament play.' *The American Journal of Sports Medicine.* 24, 279–285.

Marek, S.M., Cramer, J.T., and Culkertson, J.Y. (2005). 'Acute effects of static stretching; Effects on force and jump performance.' *Medicine and Science in Sport and Exercise.* 12, 1389–1394.

Myers, J.B., Laudner, K.G., Pasquale, M.R. *et al.* (2006). 'Glenohumeral range of motion deficits and posterior shoulder tightness in throwers with pathological internal impingement.' *The American Journal of Sports Medicine.* 34, 385–391.

Power, K. Behm, D. Cahill, M. et al. (2004). 'An acute bout of static stretching effects on force and jumping performance', *Medicine & Science in Sports and Exercise,* 83, 1389-1395.

Starrett, K. (2013). *Becoming a Supple Leopard.* Victory Belt Publishing: New Jersey, USA.

CHAPTER 4 – A FOCUS ON SHOULDER STABILITY

Baechle, T.R., and Earle, R.W. (2000). *Essentials of Strength and Conditioning Training.* Human Kinetics: Champaigne, IL.

Bak, K., and Magnusson, S.P. (1997). 'Shoulder strength and range of motion in sympathetic and pain-free elite swimmers.' *The American Journal of Sports Medicine.* 25, 454–459.

Bigliani, L.U., Rajeev, K., Pollock, R.G. *et al.* (1996). 'Glenohumeral stability: Biomechanical properties of passive and active stabilizers.' *Clinical Orthopaedics Practice.* 330, 13–30.

Burkhead, W.Z., and Rockwood, C.A. (1992). 'Treatment and instability of the shoulder with an exercise program.' *The Journal of Bone and Joint Surgery.* 74, 890–896.

Carpenter, J.E., Blasier, R.B., and Pellizzon, G.C.

(1998). 'The effects of muscle fatigue on shoulder joint position.' *The American Journal of Sports Medicine.* 42, 2–7.

Dark, A., Ginn, K.A., and Halaki, M. (2007). 'Shoulder muscle recruitment patterns during commonly used rotator cuff exercises: An electromyography study.' *Physical Therapy.* 87, 1039–1046.

Fleck, S. (2004). *Designing resistance training programs.* Human Kinetics: Champaign, IL.

Kibler, B.W. (1998). 'The use of the scapula in athletic function.' *The American Journal of Sports Medicine.* 2, 325–337.

Lloyd, R., and Oliver, J. (2012). 'The youth physical model – a new approach to long term athlete development.' *Journal of Strength and Conditioning.* 34, 61–72.

McGill, S. (2009). *Ultimate back fitness and performance.* Backfitpro Inc.: Ontario, Canada.

Prokopy, M.P., Ingersoll, C.D., Nordenchild, E. (2008). 'Closed kinetic chain upper body training improves throwing performance of NCAA division 1 softball players.' *Journal of Strength and Conditioning Research.* 12, 123 – 129.

Siff, M. (2003). *Supertraining.* Supertraining Institute: Denver.

CHAPTER 5 – TRUNK STABILITY

Baechle, T.R., and Earle, R.W. (2000). *Essentials of Strength and Conditioning Training.* Human Kinetics: Champaigne, IL.

Brown, S., and McGill, S.M. (2008). 'How the inherent stiffness of the in vivo human trunk varies with changing magnitude of muscular activation.' *Clinical Biomechanics.* 23, 15–22.

Brown, S., and McGill, S.M. (2009). 'Transmission of muscularity generated force and stiffness between layers of the rat abdominal wall.' *SPINE.* 32, E70–E75.

Gamble, P. (2007). 'An intergrated approach to training core stability.' *Strength and Conditioning Journal.* 13, 47–56.

Lee, C.A., Kessler, C.M., and Varun, D. (1998). 'Muscle rehabilitation in haemophilia.' *Haemophilia.* 4, 532–537.

McGill, S.M. (2009). *Ultimate back fitness and performance.* Backfitpro Inc.: Ontario, Canada.

McGill, S.M., Gerier, S., Bluhm, M. *et al.* (2003). 'Previous history of LBP with work loss is related to lingering deficits in biomechanical, physiological, personal psychosocial and motor control characteristics.' *Ergonomics.* 46, 731–746.

McGill, S.M., and Norman, R.W. (1987). 'Effects of anatomically detailed erector spinae model on L4/5 disc compession and shear.' *Journal of Biomechanics.* 20, 591–600.

McGill, S.M., Norman, R.W., and Sharrat, M.T. (1990). 'The effects of an abdominal belt on trunk muscle activity and intra-abdominal pressure during squat lifts.' *Ergonomics.* 33, 147–160.

Parkinson, R.J., and Callaghan, J.P. (2009). 'The role of dynamic flexion in spine injury is altered by increasing dynamic load magnitude.' *Clinical Biomechanics.* 24, 148–154.

CHAPTER 6 – PROPRIOCEPTION AND PLYOMETRIC PERFORMANCE

Baechle, T.R., and Earle, R.W. (2000). *Essentials of Strength and Conditioning Training.* Human Kinetics: Champaign, IL.

Ball, N.B., and Schuur, J.C. (2009). 'Bilateral neuromuscular and force differences during a plyometric task.' *Journal of Strength and Conditioning Research.* 23, 1433–1441.

Bennett, R.A., and Goodwin, J. (2011). *Quantifying plyometric intensity via an acute kinetic analysis.* (Unpublished)

Bennett, R.A., Goodwin, J., and Linthorne, N. (2012). *Assessing Readiness for High Stress Plyometrics.* (Unpublished)

Collier, R. (2011). 'The rise of barefoot running.' *Canadian Medical Association Journal.* 10, E37–E38.

Cook, G. (2010). *Movement: Functional movement systems – screening, assessing, corrective strategies.* On Target Publications: USA.

De Wit, B., De Clercq, D., Aerts, P. (2000). 'Biomechanical analysis of the stance phase during barefoot and shod running.' *Journal of Biomechanics.* 33, 269–278.

Ebben, W.P., and Petushek, E.J. (2010). 'Using the reactive strength index modified to evaluate plyometric performance.' *Journal of Strength and Conditioning.* 24, 1983–1987.

Giuliani, J., Masini, B., Alitz, C. *et al.* (2011). 'Barefoot-simulating footwear associated with metatarsal stress injury in 2 runners.' *Orthopedics.* 34, E320 – W323.

Hewett, T.E., Lindenfeld, M.D., Riccobene, J.V. *et al.* (1999). 'The effect of neuromuscular training on the incidence of knee injury in female athletes.' *The American Journal of Sports Medicine.* 27, 699–703.

Hoffman, J. (2012). *NSCA's guide to program design.* Human Kinetics: Champaign, IL.

Jenkins, D.W., and Cauthon, D.J. (2011). 'Barefoot running claims and controversies: A review.' *Journal of American Podiatric Medical*

Association. 101, 231–246.

Jensen, R.L., and Ebben, W.P. (2007). 'Quantifying plyometric intensity via rate of force development, knee joint and ground reaction forces.' *Journal of Strength and Conditioning Research.* 21, 763–767.

Lieberman, D.E., Venkadesan, M., Werbel. *et al.* (2010). 'Foot strike patterns and collision forces in habitually bafrefoot vs. shod runners.' *Nature.* 463, 531–535.

Lloyd, R., and Oliver, J. (2013). *Strength and conditioning for young athletes: Science and application.* Routledge: New York.

Markovic, G., and Mikulic, P. (2010). 'Neuromusculoskeletal and performance adaptations to lower extremity plyometric training.' *Sports Medicine.* 40, 859–895.

McGuine, T.A., Greene, J.J., Best, T. *et al.* (2000). 'Balance as a predictor of ankle injuries in high school basketball players.' *Clinical Journal of Sports Medicine.* 10, 239–244.

Meylan, C., and Malatesta, D. (2010). 'Effects of in-season plyometric training within soccer practice on explosive actions of young players.' *Journal of Strength and Conditioning Research.* 23, 2605–2613.

Minetti, A., Ardigo, L., Susta, D. *et al.* (1998). 'Using leg muscles as shock absorbers: Theoretical predictions and experimental results of drop landing performance.' *Ergonomics.* 41, 1771–1791.

Myer, G.D., Ford, K.R., Brent, J.L. *et al.* (2006). 'The effects of plyometric vs. dynamic stabilization and balance training on power, balance and landing force in female athletes.' *Journal of Strength and Conditioning Research.* 20, 345–353.

Nigg, B.M. (1985). 'Loads in selected sport activities: An overview.' In: Winter, D.A., and Norman, R.W. *Biomechanics IX-B.* Human Kinetics: Champaign, IL.

Potach, D.H., and Chu, D.A. (2000). 'Plyometric training.' In: *Essentials of Strength and Conditioning training.* Baechle, T.R., and Earle, R.W. Human Kinetics: Champaign, IL.

Ricard, M.D., and Veatch, S. (1994). Effect of running speed and aerobic dance jump height on vertical ground reaction forces. *Journal of Applied Biomechanics.* 10, 14–27.

Siff, M. (2003). *Supertraining.* Supertraining Institute: Denver.

Wallace, B.J., Kernozek, T.W., White. R. *et al.* (2010). 'Quantification of vertical ground reaction forces of popular bilateral plyometric exercises.' *Journal of Strength and Conditioning Research.* 24, 207–212.

CHAPTER 7 – THE FEMALE ATHLETE

American Psychiatric Association (2000). 'Practice guideline for the treatment of patients with eating disorders.' *American Journal of Psychiatry.* 157, 1–39.

American Society of Reproductive Medicine Practice Committee (2004). 'Current evaluation of amenorrhea.' *Fertility and Sterility.* 82, 266–272.

Arendt, D.E., and Dick, R. (1995). 'Knee injury patterns among men and women in collegiate basketball and soccer: NCAA data and review of literature.' *American Journal of Sports Medicine.* 23, 694–701.

Artal, R., and O'Toole, M. (2003). 'Guidelines of the American College of obstetricians and gynaecologists for exercise during pregnancy and the postpartum period.' *British Journal of Sports Medicine.* 37, 6–12.

Baechle, T.R., and Earle, R.W. (2000). *Essentials of Strength and Conditioning Training.* Human Kinetics: Champaign, IL.

Becker, A.E., Grinspoon, S.K., Kilbanski, A. *et al.* (1999). 'Eating disorders.' *North English Journal of Medicine.* 340, 1092–1098.

Boudreau, S.N., Dwyer, M.K., Mattacola, C.G. *et al.* (2005). 'Hip muscle activation during the lunge, single leg squat and step-up-and-over exercises.' *Journal of Sport Rehabilitation.* 18, 91–103.

Buckwalter, J.G., Stanzyk, F.Z., McCleary, C.A. *et al.* (1999). 'Pregnancy, the postpartum, and steroid hormones: Effects on cognition and mood.' *Psychoneuroendocrinology.* 24, 69–84.

Caterisano, A.R.F., Moss, T.K., Pellinger, K. *et al.* (2002). 'The effects of back squat depth on the EMG activity of four superficial hip and thigh muscles.' *Journal of Strength and Conditioning Research.* 16, 428–432.

Chen, H., and Tang, Y. (1989). 'Effects of menstrual cycle on respiratory muscle function.' *American Review of Respiratory Diseases.* 140, 1359–1362.

Croisier, J.L., Ganteaume, P.T., Binet, J. *et al.* (2008). 'Strength imbalances and prevention of hamstring injury in professional soccer players.' *American Journal of Sports Medicine.* 36, 1469–1475.

Filicori, M.C., Tabarelli, P., Casadio, P. (1998). 'Interaction between menstrual cyclicity gonadotropin pulsatility.' *Hormonal Research.* 49, 169–172.

Greeves, J.P., Cable, T.N., Luckas, M.J.M. *et al.* (1997). 'Effects of acute changes in oestrogen on muscle function on the first dorsal interosseus muscle in humans.' *Journal of Physiology.* 500, 265–270.

Hausmann, M., Slabberkoon, D., Van Goozen, S.H.M. *et al.* (2000). 'Sex hormones affect spatial abilities during the menstrual cycle.' *Behavioral Neuroscience.* 114, 1245–1250.

Hewett, T.E., Lindenfeld, M.D., Riccobene, J.V. *et al.* (1999). 'The effect of neuromuscular training on the incidence of knee injury in female athletes.' *The American Journal of Sports Medicine.* 27, 699–703.

Hewett, T.E., Stroupe, T.A., Nance, T.A. *et al.* (1996). 'Plyometric training in female athletes. Decreased impact forces and increased hamstring torques.' *American Journal of Sports Medicine.* 24, 765–773.

Horton, M.G., and Hall, T.L. (1989). 'Quadriceps femoris muscle angle: Normal values and relationships with gender and skeletal measures.' *Physical Therapy.* 897–901.

Hutchinson, M.R., and Ireland, M.L. (1995). 'Knee injuries in female athletes.' *Sports Medicine.* 19, 288–302.

Jansen de Jorge, X.A.K., Boot, C.R.L., Thom, J.M. *et al.* (2001). 'Influence of menstrual cycle phase on skeletal muscle contraction characteristics in humans.' *The Journal of Physiology.* 530, 161–166.

Kimura, D. (1992). 'Sex differences in the brain.' *Scientific American.* 267, 118–125.

Landgren, B.M.,Unden, A.L., and Diczfalusy, E. (1980). 'Hormonal profile of the cycle in 68 normally menstruating women.' *Acta Endocrinology.* 94, 89–90.

Laughlin, G.A., and Yen, S.S.C. (1996). 'Nutitional and endocrine-metabolic aberrations in amenorrheic athletes.' *Journal of Clinical Endocrinology and Metabolism.* 81, 301–4309.

Lebrun, C.M., McKenzie, D.C., Prior, J.C. *et al.* (1994). 'Effects of menstrual cycle phase on athletic performance.' *Medicine and Science in Sports and Exercise.* 12, 437–441.

Loucks, A.B., and Thuma, J.R. (2003). 'Luteinizing hormone pulsatility is disrupted at a threshold of energy availability in regularly menstruating women.' *Journal of Clinical Endocrinology and Metabolism.* 88, 297–311.

Mandelbaum, B.R., Silvers, H.J., Watanabe, D.S. *et al.*, (2005). Effectiveness of a neuromuscular and proprioceptive training program in preventing the incidence of anterior cruciate ligament injuries in females. 2 year follow up. *The American Journal of Sports Medicine.* 33, 1–8.

McShane, T.M., and Wise, P.M. (1996). 'Lifelong moderate caloric restriction prolongs reproductive life span in rats without interrupting estrus cyclicity: Effects on gonadotropin release hormone/luteinizing hormone axis.' *Biology and Reproduction.* 54, 70–75.

Mosekilde, L., Thompson, J.S., Orhii, P.B. *et al.* (1999). 'Addictive effect of voluntary exercise and growth hormone treatment on bone strength assessed at four different skeletal sites in an aged rat model.' *Bone.* 24, 71–80.

Myer, G.D., Ford, K.R., Brent, J.L. *et al.* (2006). 'The effects of plyometric vs. dynamic stabilization and balance training on power, balance, and landing force in female athletes.' *Journal of Strength and Conditioning Research.* 20, 345–353.

National Institutes of Health Consensus Developmental Panel (2001). 'Osteoporosis prevention, diagnosis, and therapy.' *JAMA.* 285, 785–795.

Nattiv, A., Loucks, A.B. *et al.* (2007). 'The Female Athlete Triad.' American College of Sports Medicine: *Medicine and Science in Sports and Exercise.* 1867–1882.

Noyes, F.R., Mooar, P.A., Matthews, D.S. *et al.* (1983). 'The symptomatic anterior cruciate-deficient knee. Part 1: The long term functional disability in athletically active individuals.' *Journal of Bone and Joint Surgery.* 65, 154–162.

Olsen, O.E., Mykleburst, G., Engerbresten, L. *et al.* (2005). 'Exercises to prevent lower limb injuries in youth sports.' *British Medical Journal.* 330, 1–7.

Prior, J.C., and Vigna, Y.M. (1991). 'Ovulation disturbances and exercise training.' *Clinical Obstetrics and Gynecology.* 34, 180–190.

Prior, J.C., Vigna, Y.M., Alojao, N. *et al.* (1987). 'Determination of luteal phase length by quantitative basal temperature methods: Validation against mid-cycle LH peak.' *Clinical Investigation of Medicine.* 13, 123–131.

Rome, E.S., Ammerman, S., Rosen, D.S., *et al.* (2003). 'Children and adolescents with eating disorders: The state of the art.' *Pediatrics.* 111, 98–108.

Sarwar, R., Beltran, N.B., and Rutherford, O.M. (1996). 'Changes in muscle strength, relaxation rate and fatiguability during the human menstrual cycle.' *Journal of Physiology.* 12, 23–30.

Schneider, J.E., and Wade, G.N. (2000). 'Inhibition of reproduction in service of energy balance.' In: Wallen, K. and Schneider, J.E. (2000). *Reproduction in context: Social and environmental influences on reproductive physiology and behaviour.* MIT Press: Cambridge.

Siff, M. (2003). *Supertraining.* Supertraining Institute: Denver.

Stager, J.M., Wigglesworth, J.K. and Hatler, L.K. (1990). 'Interpreting the relationship between age of menarche and prepubertal training.' *Medicine and Science in Sports and Exercise.* 22, 54–58.

Van Ingen Schenau, G.J., Bobbert, M.F., and Rozendal, R.H. (1987). 'The unique action of bi-articular muscles in complex movements.' *Journal of Anatomy.* 155, 1–5.

Vollman, R.F. (1977). 'The menstrual cycle.' In: Friedman, E.A., *Major Problems in Obstetrics and Gynecology.* W.B. Saunders: Toronto.

Wade, G.N., and Jones, J.E. (2004). 'Neuroendocrinology of nutritional fertility.' *American Journal of Physiology.* 287, 1277–1296.

Wade, G.N., Schneider, J.E., and Li, H.Y. (1996). 'Control of fertility by metabolic cues.' *American Journal of Physiology.* 270, 1–19.

Warren, M.P. (1980). 'The effect of exercise on pubertal progression and reproductive function in girls.' *Journal of Clinical Endocrinology and Metabolism.* 51, 1150–1157.

Williams, N.I., Caston-Balderama, A.L., Helmereich, D.B. *et al.* (2001). 'Longitudinal changes in reproductive hormones and menstrual cyclicity in cynomolgus monkeys during strenuous exercise training: Abrupt transition to exercise-induced amenorrhea.' *Endocrinology.* 142, 2381–2389.

Williams, N.I., Helmreich, D.L., Parfitt, D.B. *et al.* (2001). 'Evidence for a causal role of low energy availability in the induction of menstrual cycle disturbances during strenuous exercise training.' *Journal of Clinical Endocrinology and Medicine.* 86, 5184–5193.

CHAPTER 8 – MATURING AND YOUTH ATHLETES

Bahr, R. (2014). 'Demise of the fittest: are we destroying our biggest talents?' *British Journal of Sports Medicine.* 48, 1265–1267.

Baker, D., Mitchell, J., Boyle, D., *et al.* (2011). 'Resistance training for children and youth: A position stand from the Australian S&C Association.' Available at http://www.strengthandconditioning.org

Balyi, I., and Hamilton, A. (2004). *Long term athlete development: Trainability in children and adolescents; windows of opportunity.* National Coaching Institute: Canada.

Baquet, G., Van Praagh, E., and Berthoin, S. (2003). 'Endurance training and aerobic fitness in young people.' *Sports Medicine.* 33, 1127–1143.

Behm, D.G., Faigenbaum, A.D., Flak, B. *et al.* (2008). 'Exercise physiology position paper: Resistance training in children and adolescents.' *Applied Physiology, Nutrition and Metabolism.* 33, 547–561.

Behringer, M., Vom Heede, A., Matthews, M. *et al.* (2011). 'Effects of strength training on motor performances in children and adolescents: A meta-analysis.' *Paediatric Exercise Science.* 23, 18–206.

Behringer, M., Vom Heede, A., Yue, Z., *et al.* (2010). 'Effects of resistance training in children: A meta-analysis.' *Paediatrics.* 126, 1199–1210.

Beunen, G.P., and Malina, R.M. (2005). 'Growth and biological maturation: Relevance to athletic training.' In: Bar-Or, O. *The Child and Adolescent Athlete.* Blackwell Publishing: Oxford, UK.

Bloom, B.S. (1985). *Developing Talent in Young People.* Ballantine Books: New York.

Borms, J. (1986). 'The child and exercise: An overview.' *Journal of Sports Science.* 4, 4–20.

Chow, J.Y., Davids, K., Button, C. *et al.* (2008). 'Non-linear pedagogy: Implications for teaching games for understanding (TGfU).' In: *TGfU: Simply good pedagogy: Understanding a complex challenge.* University of British Columbia: Vancouver.

Clark, E.M., Tobias, J.H., Murray, L. *et al.* (2011). 'Children with low muscle strength are at an increased risk of fracture with exposure to exercise.' *Journal of Musculoskeletal Neurological Interaction.* 11, 196–202.

Comfort, P., Stewart, A., Bloom, L. *et al.* (2014). 'Relationship between strength, speed, and jump performance in well trained youth soccer players.' *Journal of Strength and Conditioning Research.* 28, 173–178.

Deli, E., Bakle, I., and Zachopoulou, E. (2006). 'Implementing intervention movement programs for kindergarten children.' *Journal of Early Child Research.* 4, 5–18.

DiFiori, J. (1999). 'Overuse injuries in children and adolescents.' *The Physician and Sports Medicine.* 27, 1–8.

Faigenbaum, A.D., Kraemer, W.J., Blimkie, C.J. *et al.* (2009). 'Youth resistance training: Updated position stand from the NSCA.' *Journal of Strength and Conditioning Research.* 23, 60–79.

Higgs, C., Balyi, I., War, R. *et al.* (2008). *Developing physical literacy: A guide for parents of chidren aged 0–12.* Canadian Sports Centre: Vancouver.

Hoff, J., Helgerud, J., and Wisloff, U. (1999). 'Maximal strength training improves work economy in trained female cross country skiers.' *Medicine and Science in Sports and Exercise.* 31, 870–877.

Jeffreys, I. (2007). 'Warm up revisited – the 'ramp' method of optimising performance preparation.' *UKSCA Journal.* 6, 15–19.

Lloyd, R.S., and Oliver, J.L. (2012). 'The Youth Physical Development Model: A new approach to long term athletic development.' *National Strength and*

Conditioning Association. 34, 61–72.

Lloyd, R., Brewer, C., Faigenbaum, A.D., *et al.* (2012). 'UKSCA position statement on youth resistance training.' *UKSCA Journal.*

Malina, R.M. (2007). 'Growth, maturation and development: Application to young athletes and in particular, to divers.' In: Malina, R.M., and Gabriel, J.L. *USA Diving Coach Development Reference Manual.* USA Diving: Indianapolis, USA.

Mirwald, R.L., Baxter-Jones, A.D., Bailey, D.A. *et al.* (2002). 'An assessment of maturity from anthropometric measurements.' *Medicine and Science in Sports and Exercise.* 34, 689–694.

Miyaguchi, K., and Demura, S. (2008). 'Relationships between muscle power output using the stretch shortening cycle and eccentric maximum strength.' *Journal of Strength and Conditioning Research.* 22, 1735–1741.

Negrete, R., and Brophy, J. (2000). 'The relationship between isokinetic open and closed kinetic chain lower extremity strength and functional performance.' *Journal of Sports Rehab.* 9, 46–61.

Newell, K.M. (1986). 'Constraints on the development of co-ordination.' In: Wage, M.G. and Whiting, T.A. *Motor development in children: Aspects of coordination and control.* Dordrecht: Netherlands.

Oliver, J.L., Lloyd, R., and Meyers, R.W. (2011). 'Training elite child athletes: Welfare and wellbeing.' *Journal of Strength and Conditioning Research.* 33, 73–79.

Philippaerts, R.M., Vaeyens, R., Janssens, M. *et al.* (2006). 'The relationship between peak height velocity and physical performance in youth soccer players.' *Journal of Sports Science.* 24, 221–230.

Santos, E., and Janeira, M.A. (2008). 'Effects of complex training on explosive strength in adolescent male basketball players.' *Journal of Strength and Conditioning Research.* 22, 903–909.

Sherar, L., Mirwald, R., Adam, G. *et al.* (2005). 'Prediction of adult height using maturity-based cumulative height velocity curves.' *The Journal of Paediatrics.* 12, 508–514.

Teeple, J.B., Lohman, T.G., Misner, J.E. *et al.* (1975). 'Contribution of physical development and muscular strength to the motor performance capacity of 7- to 12-year-old boys.' *British Journal of Sports Medicine.* 9, 122–129.

Viru, A., Loko, J., Harro, M. *et al.* (1999). 'Critical periods in the development of performance capacity during childhood and adolescence.' *European Journal of Physical Education.* 4, 75–119.

Weyand, P.G., Sternilight, D.B., Bellizzi, M.J. *et al.* (2000). 'Faster top running speeds are achieved with greater ground forces not more rapid leg movements.' *Journal of Applied Physiology.* 89, 1991–1999.

Wisloff, U., Castanga, C., Helgerud, J. *et al.* (2004). 'Strong correlations of maximal squat strength with sprint performance and vertical jump height in elite soccer players.' *British Journal of Sports Medicine.* 38, 285–288.

CHAPTER 9 – THE PHYSIOLOGY MODULE

Sleep

Atkinson, G., and Reilly, T. (1996). 'Circadian variation in sports performance.' *Sports Medicine.* 21, 292–312.

Reilly, T. (2006). *Science of training: Soccer, a scientific approach to developing strength, speed and endurance.* Routledge; London.

Reilly, T., and Edwards, B. (2006). 'Altered sleep–wake cycles and physical performance in athletes.' *Physiology and Behaviour.* 90, 274–290.

Reilly, T., Farrelly, K., Edwards, B. *et al.*, (2005). 'Effects of time of day of performance of soccer-specific motor skills.' In: Reilly, T., Cabri, J., and Araujo, D. *Science and Football.* Routledge: London.

Reilly, T., and George, A. (1983). 'Urinary phenylethamine levels during three days of soccer play.' *Journal of Sports Sciences.* 1, 70.

Resko, J.A., and Eik-Nes, K. (1966). 'Diurnal testosterone levels in peripheral plasma of human male subjects.' *The Journal of Clinical Endocrinology and Metabolism.* 26, 83–90.

Smith, R.S., and Reilly, T. (2005). 'Athletic Performance.' In: Kushida, C. *Sleep deprivation: Clinical issues, pharmacology and sleep loss effects.* Marcel Dekker: New York.

Stampi, C., Broughton, R., Mullington, J., *et al.* (1990). 'Ultrashort sleep strategies during sustained operations: The recuperative value of 80-, 50-, and 20-min naps.' In: Costa, G., Cesana, G., Kogi, K. *et al. Shiftwork, health and sleep performance.* Peter Lang: Frankfurt.

Thomas, V. and Reilly, T. (1975). 'Circulatory, psychological and performance variables during 100 hours of continuous exercise under conditions of controlled energy intake and work output.' *Journal of Human Movement Studies.* 1, 149–155.

The stress of travel

Bor, R. (2003). *Passenger Behaviour.* Ashgate: Aldershot, UK.

Brown, T., Shuker, L., Rushton, L. *et al.* (2001). 'The possible effects on health, comfort and safety of aircraft cabin environments.' *Journal of the Royal Society for Promotion of Health.* 121, 177–184.

de Looy, A., Minors, D., Waterhouse, J. *et al.* (1988). *The Coach's Guide to Competing Abroad.* National Coaching Foundation: Leeds.

Tsai, T., Okumura, M., Yamasaki, M. *et al.* (1988). 'Simulation of jet lag following a trip with stopovers by intermittent scheduled shifts.' *Journal of Interdisciplinary Cycle Research.* 19, 89–96.

Waterhouse, J. (2001). 'Time in biology with particular reference to humans.' *European Review.* 9, 31–42.

Waterhouse, J., Reilly, T., and Edwards, B. (2004). 'The stress of travel.' *Journal of Sports Sciences.* 22, 946–966.

The stress of the heat

Davis, J.M., Alderson, N.L., and Welsh, R.S. (2000). 'Serotonin and central nervous system fatigue: nutritional considerations.' *American Journal of Clinical Nutrition.* 72, 573S–578S.

Galloway, S.D.R., and Maughan, R.J. (1997). 'Effects of ambient temperature on the capacity to perform prolonged cycle exercise in man.' *Medicine and Science in Sports and Exercise.* 29, 1240–1249.

Gonzales-Alonso, J., Calbet, J.A., and Nielsen, B. (1999). 'Metabolic and thermodynamic responses to dehydration-induced restrictions in muscle blood flow in exercising humans.' *Journal of Physiology.* 520, 577–589.

Gonzales-Alonso, J., Teller, C., Andersen, S.L. *et al.* (1999). 'Influence of body temperature on the development of fatigue during prolonged exercise in the heat.' *Journal of Applied Physiology.* 86, 1032–1039.

Maughan, R., and Shirreffs, S. (2004). 'Exercise in the heat: Challenges and opportunities.' *Journal of Sports Sciences.* 22, 917–927.

Nielsen, B., Hales, J.R., Strange, S. *et al.* (1993). 'Human circulatory and thermoregulatory adaptations with heat acclimation and exercise in a hot, dry environment.' *Journal of Physiology.* 460, 467–485.

Nielsen, B., Hyldig, T., Bidstrup, F. *et al.* (2001). 'Brain activity and fatigue during prolonged exercise in the heat.' Pflügers Archiv European *Journal of Physiology.* 442, 41–48.

Sawka, M.N., and Pandolf, K.B. (1990). 'Effects of body water loss on physiological function and exercise performance.' In: *Perspective in Sport Medicine and Exercise Science Vol. 3.* Benchmark Press: Indianapolis.

Shirreffs, S.M., Taylor, A.J., Leiper, J.B. *et al.* (1996). 'Post exercise rehydration in man: Effects of volume consumed and sodium content of ingested fluids.' *Medicine and Science in Sports and Exercise.* 28, 1260–1271.

Exercise in the cold

Doubt, T.J. (1991). 'Physiology of exercise in the cold.' *Sports Medicine.* 11, 367–381.

Epstein, Y., Shapiro, Y., and Brill, S. (1983). 'Role of surface area to mass ratio and work efficiency in heat tolerance.' *Journal of Applied Physiology.* 54, 831–836.

Faulkner, J.A., White, T.P., and Markeley, J.M. (1981). 'The 1979 Canadian ski marathon: A natural experiment in hypothermia.' In: *Exercise in health and disease.* Thomas: Springfield.

Febbraio, M.A., Snow, R.J., Sathis, C.G. *et al.* (1996). 'Blunting the rise in body temperature reduces muscle glycogenolysis during exercise in humans.' *Experimental Physiology.* 81, 685–693.

Hanna, J.M., McHill, P., Sinclair, J.D. (1975). 'Human cardiorespiratory responses to acute cold exposure.' *Clinical and Experimental Pharmacology and Physiology.* 2, 229–238.

Molnar, G.W. (1946). 'Survival of hypothermia by men immersed in the ocean.' *Journal of the American Medical Assocation.* 131, 1046–1050.

Nadel, E.R., Holmer, I., Beegh, U. *et al.* (1974). 'Energy exchanges of swimming man.' *Journal of Applied Physiology.* 36, 465–471.

Nimmo, M. (2004). 'Exercise in the cold.' *Journal of Sports Science.* 22, 898–916.

Rennie, D.W. (1988). 'Tissue heat transfer in water: Lessons from the Korean divers.' *Medicine and Science in Sports and Exercise.* 20, S177–S184.

Smith, G.B., and Hames, E.F. (1962). 'Estimation of tolerance times for cold water immersion.' *Aerospace Medicine.* 33, 834–840.

Smith, R.M., and Hanna, J.M. (1975). 'Skinfolds and resting heat loss in cold air and water: Temperature equivalence.' *Journal of Applied Physiology.* 39, 93–102.

Tipton, M.J. (1989). 'The initial responses to cold water immersion in man.' *Clinical Science.* 77, 581–588.

Tipton, M.J., Mekjavic, I.B., and Eglin, C.M. (2000). 'Permanence of the habituation of the initial responses to cold-water immersion in humans.' *European Journal of Applied Physiology.* 83, 17–21.

Toner, M.M., and McArdle, W.D. (1988). 'Physiological adjustment to man in the cold.' In: *Human Performance: Physiology and Environmental Medicine at Terrestrial Extremes.* Cooper Publishing Group: Carmel, CA.

Wagner, J.A., and Horvath, S.M. (1985). 'Influence of age and gender on human thermoregulation responses to cold exposures.' *Journal of Applied Physiology.*

Werner, J., Reents, T., (1980). 'A contribution to the topography of temperature regulation in man.' *European Journal of Applied Physiology.* 45, 87–94.

Effects of exercise on the immune function

Ekblom, B., Ekblom, O., and Malm, C. (2006). 'Infectious episodes before and after a marathon race.' *Scandinavian Journal of Medicine and Sports Science.* 16, 287–293.

Gerdhem, P., Ringsberg, K., Obrant, K. et al. (2005). 'Association between 25-hydroxy vitamin D levels, physical acitivity, muscle strength and fractures in the prospective population-based OPRA study of elderly women. *Osteoporosis.* 16, 1425–1431.

Gleeson, M. (2007). 'Immune function in sport and exercise.' *Journal of Applied Physiology.* 101, 690–699.

Matthews, C.E., Ockene, J.S., Fredson, P.S. et al. (2002). 'Moderate to vigorous physical activity and the risk of upper respiratory tract infection.' *Medicine and Science in Sport and Exercise.* 34, 1242–1248.

Nieman, D.C. (1994). 'Exercise, infection and immunity'. *International Journal of Sports Medicine.* 15, S131–S141.

Peters, E.M., Goeetzsche, J.M., Grobbelaar, B. et al. (1993). 'Vitamin C supplementation reduces the incidence of post race symptoms of upper respiratory tract infections in ultra-marathon runners.' *American Journal of Clinical Nutrition.* 57, 170–174.

Peters, E.M., Goeetzsche, J.M., Joseph, L.E. et al. (1996). 'Vitamin C as effective as combinations of anti-oxidant nutrients in reducing symptoms of URTI in ultramarathon runners.' *South African Journal of Sports Medicine.* 11, 23–27.

Pilcher, J., Gurter, D., and Sadowsky, B. (1997). 'Sleep quality versus sleep quantity: Relationships between sleep and measures of health, well-being and sleepiness in college students.' *Journal of Psychosomatic Research.* 42, 583–596.

CHAPTER 10 – REHAB FROM AN S&C PERSPECTIVE

Baker, D. (2011). 'Recent trends in high-intensity aerobic training for field sports.' *UKSCA Journal.* 22, 3–9.

Billat, L.V. (2001). 'Interval training for performance, a scientific and empirical practice. Part 2: Anaerobic interval training.' *Sports Medicine.* 31, 75–90.

Blagrove, R. (2014). 'Minimising the interference effect during programmes of concurrent strength and endurance training. Part 2: Progamming recommendations.' *UKSCA Journal.* 32, 13–20.

Buchheit, M., and Laursen, P.B. (2013). 'High intensity interval training: Solution to the programming puzzle.' *Sports Medicine.* 34, 513–538.

Chilibeck, P.D., Bell, G.J., Farrar, R.P. et al. (1998). 'Higher mitochondrial fatty acid oxidation following intermittent versus continuous endurance exercise training.' *Canadian Journal of Physiology and Pharmacology.* 76, 891–894.

Gabbet, T., Kelly, J. and Pezet, T. (2007). 'Relationship between physical fitness and playing ability in rugby league players.' *Journal of Strength and Conditioning Research.* 13, 19–27.

Girard, O., Mendez-Villanueva, A., and Bishop, D. (2011). 'Repeated sprint ability, Part 1: Factors contributing to fatigue.' *Sports Medicine.* 41, 673–694.

Green, H. J., Coates, G., Sutton, J. R. et al. (1991). 'Early adaptations in gas exchange cardiac function and haematology to prolonged exercise training in man.' *European Journal of Applied Physiology.* 63, 17–23.

Green, H.J., Jones, L.L., Houston, M.E. et al. (1989). 'Muscle energetics during prolonged cycling after hypovolemia.' *Journal of Applied Physiology.* 66, 622–631.

Green, H. J., Jones, L. L., and Painter, D. C. (1990). Effects of short term training on cardiac function during prolonged exercise. *Medicine and Science in Sport and Exercise.* 22, 488–493.

Green, H.J. (1992). 'Muscular adaptations to extreme altitude: Metabolic implications during exercise.' *International Journal of Sports Medicine.* 13, S163–S165.

Hickson, R.S., Bomze, H., and Holloszy, J. (1977). 'Linear increase in aerobic power induced by a strenuous programme of endurance exercise.' *Journal of Applied Physiology.* 42, 372–276.

Laursen, P.B., and Jenkins, D.G. (2002). 'The Scientific Basis for High Intensity Interval

Training.' *Sports Medicine.* 32, 53–73.

Lee, M., Gandevia, S., Carrol, T. (2009). 'Unilateral strength training increases voluntary activation of the opposite untrained limb.' *Clinical Neurophysiology.* 120, 802–808.

Loenneke, J.P., Wilson, G.J., Wilson, J.M. (2010). 'A mechanistic approach to blood flow occlusion.' *International Journal of Sports Medicine.* 31, 1–4.

McKenzie, S., Phillips, S., Carter, S. *et al.* (2000). 'Endurance exercise training attenuates leucine oxidation and BCOAD activation during exercise in humans.' *American Journal of Physiology, Endocrinology and Metabolism.* 278, E580–E587.

Munn, J., Herbert, R.D., and Gandevia, S. (2004). 'Contralateral effects of unilateral resistance training: A meta analysis.' *Journal of Applied Physiology.* 96, 1861–1866.

Munn, J., Herbert, R.D., Hancock, M.J. *et al.* (2005). 'Training with unilateral resistance exercise increases contralateral strength.' *Journal of Applied Physiology.* 99, 1880–1884.

Rowell, A.L. (1993). *Human Cardiovascular Control.* Oxford University Press: New York.

Shima, N., Ishida, K., Katayama, K. *et al.* (2002). Cross education of muscular strength during unilateral resistance training and detraining. *European Journal of Applied Physiology.* 86, 287–294.

Siff, M. (2004). *Supertraining.* Supertraining Institute: Denver.

Smith, D.J., Roberts, D., and Watson, B. (1992). 'Physical, physiological and performance differences between Canadian national team and university volleyball players.' *Journal of Sports Sciences.* 10, 131–138.

Tabata, I., Nishimura, K., Kouzaki, M. *et al.* (1996). 'Effects of moderate-intensity endurance and high intensity intermittent training on anaerobic capacity and VO2 max.' *Medicine and Science in Sport and Exercise.* 28, 1327–1330.

Takarada, Y., Nakamura, Y., Aruga, S. *et al.* (2000a). 'Rapid increase in plasma growth hormone after low intensity resistance exercise with vascular occlusion.' *Journal of Applied Physiology.* 88, 61–65.

Takarada, Y., Sato, Y., and Ishii, N. (2002). 'Effects of resistance exercise combined with vascular occlusion on muscle function in athletes.' *European Journal of Applied Physiology.* 86, 308–314.

Takarada, Y., Takazawa, H., Sato, Y. *et al.* (2000b). 'Effects of resistance exercise combined with moderate vascular occlusion on muscular function in humans.' *Journal of Applied Physiology.* 88, 2097–2106.

Tomlin, D.L., and Wenger, H.A. (2001). 'The relationship between aerobic fitness and recovery from high intensity intermittent exercise.' *Sports Medicine.* 31, 1–11.

Van Winckel, J., Helsen, W., and McMillan, K. *et al.* (2014). *Fitness in soccer: The science and practical application.*

Weltman, A., Snead, D., and Seip, R. (1990). 'Percentages of maximal heart rate/heart rate reserve and VO2 max for determining endurance training intensity in male runners.' *International Journal of Sports Medicine.* 11, 218–222.

Zhou, S. (2000). 'Chronic neural adaptations to unilateral exercise: Mechanisms of cross-education.' *Exercise and Sports Science Review.* 28, 177–184.

INDEX